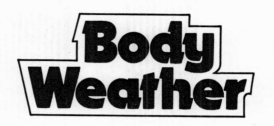

# Body Weather

## HOW NATURAL AND MAN-MADE CLIMATES AFFECT YOU AND YOUR HEALTH

### Bruce Palmer

## Stackpole Books

BODY WEATHER

Copyright © 1976 by
Bruce Palmer

Published by
STACKPOLE BOOKS
Cameron and Kelker Streets
Harrisburg, Pa. 17105

Printed in the U.S.A.

**Library of Congress Cataloging in Publication Data**

Palmer, Bruce.
  Body weather.

  Bibliography: p.
  Includes index.
    1.  Climatology, Medical. 2. Man—Influence of climate. I. Title.
RA793.P3        613.1′1        76–922
ISBN 0–8117–0245–6

# Contents

# Introduction

The weather, one way or another, is always on everybody's mind. It's probably the most popular topic of conversation there is, and for good reason: through his history man has had to adapt to climate and weather conditions as part of his environment. Our bodies evolved in intimate relation with certain temperatures, storms, light patterns, and the turn of the seasons. But today the advent of technology, and especially central heating and air conditioning, has put us in a vastly different environment most of the time; the average citizen spends only a small fraction of his time in natural weather. Cut off from the atmosphere outside temperature-controlled offices and snugly heated homes, we have forgotten how all these kinds of weather—man-made and natural—affect us. We have forgotten a primordial lesson, that the weather conditions outside, in a very real sense, determine the conditions in our minds and bodies.

Our bodies, however, have not forgotten. Evidence is increasing that today's man-made weather is subjecting the human body to stresses that it was not meant to endure, threatening the very health it was meant to promote. Air conditioning brought us summertime comfort—and the summer cold. Central heating has taken the chill out of our bones, and left us with dry throats and nasal membranes. What we have forgotten, it seems, is that our bodies evolved in response to *natural* weather conditions. And while we have engineered climate control, we did not engineer the human body.

Of course, man must live with his technology. But first and foremost, he must learn to live with his own body, and that body was designed to respond to weather conditions. Not surprisingly, those pretechnological conditions often turn out to be more healthy than the artificial ones prevailing today. There is abundant evidence, for example, that long-wave ultraviolet rays in full-spectrum sunlight (usually filtered out through windowglass) have a therapeutic value for the treatment of many diseases, including cancer, arthritis, and psoriasis. And in fact, we can use an enlightened technology to complement human biology. Fluorescent light bulbs which approximate full-spectrum light are now available, and where they have been installed, workers' productivity has soared. Windows of ultraviolet-transmitting glass have produced a similar effect.

The purpose of this book is to make available to the general reader the best information on how the human body and mind are affected by the impacts of climate, weather, wind, light, and noise— and to make suggestions about new ways of using modern technology intelligently to find appropriate ways of responding to the stresses of modern life. *Body Weather* is really a key to understanding and controlling your own intimate weather.

# 1

# Climates, Weather, and Human Health

The humorist Mark Twain observed that humans have a single topic of conversation in common. "Everybody complains about the weather," he wrote, "but nobody does anything about it." Yet, at his new home in Hartford, Connecticut, Twain could press a button and turn night into day with his modern electric light system, the very latest thing. Down in the basement, a family servant flung a shovelful of coal into the furnace, and the writer's study was comfortably warmed in midwinter. On summer afternoons, canvas awnings shaded his veranda, as deep as the deck on a Mississippi steamboat, and cooled his bedroom, while a hose sprinkled Twain's lawn, nourishing the grass and lowering the temperature of the air he breathed. If the needle on the barometer hanging in the front hall dropped, Mark Twain reached for his umbrella. His quip was a half-truth, for man, since he first used fire to warm a cave, has regularly tried to "do something" about the weather. In large measure, he has been able to make the spaces and places where he works, plays, and rests not only more convenient, but more comfortable. In the last few decades, medical scientists as well as meteorologists have become certain that climate, both natural and artificial, affects human health. As we have learned to do something about the weather, it is now possible to know that the weather does something, day and night, to us.

In Shakespeare's play, the Scots general Macbeth comes on stage after a great and bloody victory. He is a national hero, the savior of the kingdom. What does he say? "So foul and fair a day I have not seen." Typical Britisher, chatting about the weather. Why, yes, we have driven out the invaders and crushed a rebellion, but on the other hand, it looks rather like we might be in for a spot of rain. Although it was patriotic to claim that brave British seadogs had driven off the Spanish Armada, most Englishmen of Shakespeare's day could remember that the worst storm in thirty years had battered and wrecked the enemy invasion fleet off the Irish coast.

Three hundred and forty-six years later, General Dwight Eisenhower might have had reason to recall another famous line of verse: "What is so rare as a day in June?" The mighty fleet, poised to invade France, waited and waited. The most important decision made on D-Day was approval for sailing, issued by the Allied commander's chief meteorological officer, the weatherman. Then, as earlier, the weather was "the alpha and omega of British conversation," as the wit Thomas Love Peacock put it. Realistically, climate conditions as facts of life have played important parts in the development of man. Artistically, the weather has often been employed as symbolic of internal states of being, both physical and mental. Scientifically, climate and weather can now be observed with considerable accuracy, predictions made on the basis of accumulated data, and measurements made of their effect on the total health of man.

In the past half-century, technologists and life-scientists have devoted hundreds of thousands of man-hours and millions of research and development dollars to the task of gaining a larger measure of control over the conditions that affect living creatures: plants, animals, and man. Some of their work has changed our weather, at least locally. Other by-products of technology seem to have altered, slightly, the climate of some temperate areas or to have contributed enough to natural climate change that we are somewhat more aware of certain phenomena. Overall, we are better informed, since our globe is now circled by artificial satellites that monitor, map, and transmit information about the natural forces and conditions that encourage or threaten life. We have even learned to "make" weather, at least to the degree of increasing our own level of comfort, regardless of seasonal change.

Air conditioners and humidifiers cool and modify the temperature and moisture of offices, schools, private homes, buses, and automobiles. The same systems can convert subtropical conditions to temperate comfort, thus altering the geographical distribution of humans and increasing their productivity. Human ingenuity has made it possible for people to live in the Antarctic, underwater, and in airless space. Because work, study, transportation, recreation, and rest have been made easier, our lives can be more productive, less exhausting, and measurably healthier. We have also learned, however, that this is not always the case, for every convenience and comfort may affect us in ways we neither anticipated nor want. By deliberate acts designed to change the inconvenient to the comfortable, we have unintentionally created new health hazards.

Economics is involved, not only in air-conditioned factories and offices where comfortable employees produce more goods and services faster, but in those controlled spaces and places where humans play or pay to watch others perform. Huge enclosed sports arenas like the Astrodome in Houston, Texas provide near-perfect conditions, day and night. Spectators, certain of comfort and sure that no contest will be cancelled, are ready customers. Good weather, natural or controlled, is good for business and the business of recreation. The Romans roofed their Colosseum with canvas. (The word "arena" comes from the Latin for "sand," the first artificial playing surface.) Ironically, there is enough sheer mass of air inside modern sports facilities to permit condensation of moisture in the form of rain, even when the weather outside is clear!

If by economy we mean the prudent utilization of resources for survival or gain, an examination of the undesired effects of climate control may suggest that overutilization of the new technology harms us as much as it helps us. Some observers believe that the changes made for convenience and comfort involve paying a stiff price in human physical and mental health. But before we consider the impacts of the artificial, an examination of the natural is in order.

## NATURAL CLIMATE, NATURAL WEATHER, AND NATURAL MAN

### Rainfall

The vital substance of life on the earth is water. We have learned to prevent rain from falling on a sports surface in Texas and have been able to "seed" some cloud formations in other locales to cause rain to fall there, not elsewhere. This control is not perfect; not everything man attempts always works. In Israel and Arizona, water diverted by irrigation systems has converted vast tracts of desert to arable land. The new plant-life, in turn, cools the air above it, easing life for animals and man. Add water to the earth and life will change. The weather will change, too. In another area, Central Africa, the Sahara is drifting south, altering its position by about 15 degrees in latitude. There, man is helpless, and the results of change are not local but global. The belt of monsoons, periodic heavy rains, has shifted, altering plant, animal, and human life. Recent magazine articles and television documentaries have made us aware that millions in Africa and Asia face starvation. Despite man's capacity to create infields and apple orchards or to make pastures from dust bowls, nature still embraces us all in her indifferent clasp. Too little water destroys plants, cattle, and children in the Sudan; an astonishing excess of water and wind brushes the continent of Australia and destroys the city of Darwin in a few terrifying minutes. Generally speaking, the smaller the area and the shorter the time involved, the better man's control can be. Closed air spaces can be managed with a certain degree of efficiency for practical or frivolous use. Limited open areas are controllable for limited times. The major modifications of life remain natural in cause and seem likely to remain so for many generations. We have gained somewhat in application, more in education.

### Ecology and Biometeorology

The schools, colleges, and universities of many technologically advanced nations now offer courses of study in ecology, the scientific investigation of the relationships between living things and their environments. Elementary school children in Europe, America, and Japan learn to understand the concepts of ecosystems and biotics and to dislike the impact of earth, water, and air pollution on humans. "Ecology," a new word, comes from the ancient Greek *oikos*, meaning "house." When we study how life can be altered, improved, damaged, or destroyed by man-made changes in the environments surrounding or enclosing complex systems, we are learning a new form of economics, a kind of prudent resource-use that is "housekeeping." The concept "Spaceship Earth" has become almost a cliché; yet the phrase does help to remind us that our planet is the home of life, at least as we now know it. Our imaginative awareness of our world has begun to change, although we seem to prefer to maintain those habits we have learned to think of as "natural." By this, we sometimes mean symptomatic of technology rather than associated with nature.

A smaller but growing number of research specialists and medical scientists in this country, Asia, and Europe have devoted their careers, time, energy, and money to examining the relationship between man and his environment, but with the emphasis reversed. They have learned a good deal about how natural environments affect humans, animals, and plants and have considered the impacts of artificial environments as well. Once called "medical climatology," the field has a new name: "biometeorology." If we have come to recognize, perhaps in the nick of time, that we must keep our house, then we should want to know more about how our house keeps us.

As we control, to some significant degree, the weather and the climate of our natural environment, so we are controlled or changed, both physically and mentally, by the climate and the weather of this same environment. A look at man's history may make it easier to see that *how* man lives is determined by *where* he lives. It is more simple to consider the discomforts of the past than the convenience of the present in order to grasp the significance of the new sciences. The superstitions, habits, and customs of one's ancestors are so obviously silly that we are able to forget the follies of our own time. If we reflect, though, on the fact that our technology has reversed living conditions to the point that we live, most of the time, within artificial climates and weathers, then we may be willing to grant that in the process of creating comforts unknown to the past, we have developed dangers previously undreamed of. Convenience? Without question. Health hazards? Without question, too. We want the former without the latter, but don't always get it. Sometimes, we seem to get the reverse.

To answer Mark Twain, we *can* and we *do* change the weather. Like Macbeth, we have come to understand that what seems fair may prove to be foul, and vice versa. One definition has told us for generations that educated man knows what he knows, while a wise man knows what he knows and also what he does *not* know. The new scientific fields of ecology and biometeorology are presently expanding the totals of both human knowledge and human wisdom. What may prove surprising is that apparently simple factors may be affecting our physical and mental health in both large and small ways every day. We can alter and "improve" our environments locally, but we cannot escape the impacts of larger forces ever.

## Climate and Weather Defined

Among these larger forces that influence, for better or worse, our physical and mental health are climate and weather. We need a clear distinction between them. While climate and weather have comparable effects of the human body, the two are not the same thing and should not be thought of as approximate synonyms or even roughly interchangeable terms.

Climate is considered to be the *average* of conditions of temperature, wind speed and wind direction, atmospheric pressure, and humidity *over long periods of time*. Climate can be measured by the year, but is more accurately described on the basis of observations taken over decades. Outside tropical zones, temperature, atmospheric pressure, wind speed, and rainfall vary greatly. The average of each factor, calculated over forty years, a working lifetime, may appear much more stable. There have been significant changes in climate in the historical past. That is, the averages themselves have altered. During the Dark Ages, wine grapes grew in England and Norse settlers harvested grain in Iceland. The climate was warmer. All of Europe was warmer, on the average, 1,000 years ago than it has been, on the average, since that time.

Weather is *measured* conditions of temperature, wind speed and wind direction, atmospheric pressure, and humidity *at a given time*. That is, weather can be thought of as short-term climate: "The weather has been pretty good, for November." More commonly, weather is thought of in week-long segments, since adverse conditions are likely to effect changes in scheduled or anticipated work and recreation. Most of us think of the weather as the sum of phenomena day by day or "what it's doing out" right now. Millions listen to or watch radio and television weathermen. Climate-persons do not exist for most of us.

Climate is not predicted as a public service, while the weather is. That man inside the box said it would snow and now it's raining. Weathermen are notoriously "wrong," so far as the inconvenienced public is concerned. Actually, weather predictions are generally accurate on the average, for that is what the meteorologist employs in his forecasts: averages and means, the typical or usual. When a dozen or so conditions approximate those recorded on a clear day, the chances are four to one that tomorrow will approximate quite closely the other clear days of the given season. Predictions are not prophecies, but estimates about a given period based on information collected in the past. The long sum of weather makes a climate, while the records kept on a climate enable us to estimate the next day's weather.

Consider the predicted snow that fell as rain. We tend to forget that all large cities radiate enormous amounts of heat, enough to melt a moderate snowfall hundreds of feet above the pavement and rooftops. The meteorologist's forecast was correct, and so was our experience. Nobody made any mistake. An artificial condition affected a natural phenomenon, a situation more common in metropolitan areas than in rural sections.

The sum of atmospheric conditions is made of many variables: air temperature and atmospheric pressure; wind velocity and direction; the degree of moisture and type of actual or estimated precipitation (rain, sleet, snow, hail); type, altitude, and thickness of cloud cover; the position of the earth in relation to the sun; the time-length of exposure to solar radiation as the earth turns on its axis; the location of the moon in relation to the earth and the sun; the gain or loss of electrical charges in the atmosphere; the size of land or water mass, and altitude above sea-level—to name the most obvious. All of these natural factors can and do change widely over relatively brief time spans. In fact, weather *becomes* more than weather *is*. The weather, anywhere on the surface of the earth, is always becoming colder, darker, drier, windier, sunnier, moonier or warmer, brighter, wetter and so forth without end. Since we are exposed to weather— that is, conditions in a state of continuous change—humans are constantly changing also, reacting dramatically or subtly, consciously or not, in body, mind, and spirit.

The amount of weather man experiences today, however, is almost the reverse of that endured or enjoyed by his ancestors. In the pretechnological era of the Dark Ages, the European worked, played, and lived generally in the open, rising with the sun and resting at nightfall. His buildings provided only shelter and work-space during inclement conditions. Artificial light was limited. Artificial heat was limited, too, with wood and peat as the principal fuels. Now, the European goes out of doors very little, usually in travel to and from work. The artificial heating and lighting of his shelters and work-space permits their use night and day, regardless of season. Bad weather is a nuisance, an inconvenience to modern man; good weather is largely irrelevant. It is not surprising, then, that contemporary humans are accustomed, not to climate and weather, but to ignoring both and discounting both as conditioning or controlling factors of life. No longer the slave of the seasons, modern man scarcely notes their passage.

15

As we shall see, this reversal, wherein the artificial has replaced the natural as the standard environment, means not that we are "free" but rather that we react, physically and mentally, to artifice. We may have worked to eliminate inconvenience and discomfort, but we have not succeeded in eliminating our reflexes and responses to stimuli. We can make an environment that is totally artificial, a windowless box enclosing air of constant temperature, humidity level, and pressure. So long as we choose or are forced to wake and sleep, work, and rest within it, just so long will our bodies and minds react to it. Predictably, our physical and mental health will suffer. A maximum security prison is such an environment, or nearly so. We do not employ such structures as health resorts.

### Nature's Rhythm of Light and Dark

The prisoner in the cell and the laboratory animal in its cage are extreme examples of life in controlled environments. Despite existences deprived of most natural influences, however, the convict and the white rat will react and respond to fluctuations of atmospheric pressure and to other regular rhythms of life caused by the peculiarities of the planet.

Life is fastened by gravity to a distorted sphere, a bit flat at each pole, tilted slightly off the perpendicular and bulged in the Southern Hemisphere. Our planet spins west to east as it moves in its orbit around the sun at approximately 1,000 miles per hour. We do not feel that we rush through space, but cannot fail to notice the day-to-night changes that occur as the particular spot we are glued to turns to expose us to the sun's light and heat, then rolls on and away, carrying us back into darkness. We know that the sun only seems to rise and set. Actually, it is revealed and then concealed in a recurring rhythm of life.

Our position on the globe, as measured in miles from the equator, constitutes one of the conditions of climate, weather, and health. Our position, calculated in feet above sea level, constitutes another condition and encourages heightened awareness. The day-night change is intense on a mountaintop because of the altitude and in the desert, too, since in both locations sudden changes from light to darkness and back are accompanied by rapid cooling and heating. This alternating pattern of light and dark, with accompanying rise and fall of air temperature, is called the *diurnal rhythm* and affects all forms of life. Activity of animals and people varies in degree and kind, but does not cease. We all know "day people" and "night people," those whose activities slow at twilight and those who seem to waken very slowly but seem to function well after dark. There is some seasonal variation in the diurnal rhythm of each individual, and our days and nights can be reversed under artificial conditions that retrain both the body and the mind.

Scientists—who point out that the elapsed time we call a "day" lasts 24.0 hours, 24.8 hours, or 23.9 hours, depending on whether the space-object used to measure the rotation of the earth is the sun, the moon, or a fixed star—prefer the word "circadian" which means (surprisingly casual for scientists) "about a day long" when referring to daily body rhythms. *Circadian rhythms* are uniform, under normal circumstances, regardless of a person's physical position on the globe. A Canadian, Chilean, or Chinese has the same circadian rhythm, or very nearly so with other persons his same age. Anyone who has raised a child knows that an infant's circadian rhythm differs from that of an adult. Once past youth, however, humans can be said to experience the same weather-per-day in terms of day-to-night alternation, regardless of climate.

## Natural Wind Patterns

The speed and direction of the wind is one of the constantly changing conditions that make up the total of weather, which in turn affects human well-being and impinges on human awareness. We are more conscious of our physical mass when a breeze strokes or a gale buffets our bodies. Wind and temperature combine to produce a measurable "chill factor," often given with the morning and evening news and weather predictions. Such facts increase our mental sensitivity. We claim to feel colder if provided with measurements. Wind, temperature, and water in the form of vapor combine to make clouds, also a weather condition. By blocking the rays of light and heat from the sun, clouds affect air temperature on or near the surface of the earth.

What causes the wind? Surprisingly few people know. Most people believe that air causes the wind. Actually, this apparently simple fact of nature is the end result of the changing relationship in space between the earth and its moon. Like other natural phenomena, it is not quite so simple as one might first suppose. Wind is a mass of air moving in a circular direction. The movement around *low*-pressure centers (counterclockwise in the Northern, clockwise in the Southern Hemisphere) is a *cyclone* pattern. If the air mass swirls around *high*-pressure centers (clockwise in the Northern

Hemisphere, counterclockwise in the Southern), this is an *anticyclone* pattern. Both conditions are quite normal and are created by water. Cyclones and anticyclones move hundreds and even thousands of miles, changing direction and varying in speed.

### Moon, Tide, and Wind

Our planet attracts the moon with enough force to keep it in orbit, while the moon is, in turn, large enough and close enough to the earth to exert force upon the water that covers about two-thirds of the surface of our planet. The moon plucks or tugs on the water turned closest to it as the earth rotates. The oceans are pulled out, toward the moon, then gradually released as the exposed side of our planet turns away. The moon circles the earth, of course, completing an orbit every 27.3 days, but does not rotate on its own axis, thus showing the same face to all earth dwellers. The moon-dwellers of the future will be able to watch the entire surface of the earth in rotating exposure every 24.8 hours. The waters of our spinning planet, once tugged toward the moon, continue to surge in that direction as a tide, reaching a high point on land in the way of their motion. High tide changes daily, occurring forty-eight minutes later each day at the same spot.

While all this is going on, the moon also pulls on the atmosphere of gases that encloses and protects life on our globe. Like the oceans, the portion of the atmosphere closest to the moon is pulled. Then, as the earth rotates, the force is lessened. The atmosphere, in this way, is made to flow or surge, rather like the tides. As the depth of ocean touching a given spot rises and falls, so the atmosphere over that spot has a high and low tide. Both ocean depth and depth of atmosphere exist in states of continuous change, always becoming a condition. As the gross amount of air above us is tugged or released, so its weight or pressure upon us rises and falls. Given the spin of the earth and the vastness of distance and force, not all areas of air or ocean can be affected at any given time or equally. The air above certain sections or zones of the earth has atmospheric pressure that tends to be consistently high; the air above other areas has prevailing low pressure. Air tends to flow like water; the capacity to be moved is one of the characteristics of air. Pulled and released by the moon, air whirls, clockwise or counterclockwise, rather like water swirling down a bathtub drain.

Given the regularity of the orbits of moon and earth, it would seem that the creation of wind should be standard, hence predictable. Yet the weather maps or radar patterns shown on the home television screen often look like huge, whirling disturbances on the prowl or long walls sweeping over the continent, very much like the "front" of an invading army. As planets go, the earth is relatively smooth, with ancient upheavals of rock eroded by water action and wind-blown dirt. Locally, however, the planet is irregular enough to deflect cyclone or anticyclone air. Smaller, regional topographic features such as a large inland lake, modest mountains, or broad, flat plains alter air direction and amount of water vapor, the factors that dominate the weather in any given locality. Because of regional geography affecting the surge and decline of ocean and atmospheric depth, high and low pressure centers do not have permanently fixed locations or totally predictable rhythms. Weather is not uniformly distributed, as we all know, but many local variations from the norm are possible and stated to us as "unseasonably hot (cold) (dry) (rainy)."

## The Seasons

The seasons themselves, traditionally divided into four, are approximates of time, each containing quite wide differences in the abruptness and frequency of change. Weather, while inescapable, is the least uniform and most unpredictable factor of the modern environment. Seasons, determined by the direction of the axis of our tilted earth in its annual trip around the sun, are typical. It is climate that is best described as "average," since it is calculated from the midpoints of range in more than a dozen conditions.

## Climate as a Cultural Factor

Anthropologists are generally agreed that climate is a major determining factor as to what a group, tribe, nation, or race may accomplish over long periods of time. Climate affects culture, then. Weather, variable by region and locale, influences all humans equally only insofar as they all get the same amount. Certainly they do not get the same kind. The unequal distribution and the kind of weather we get affects us unequally, day by day, hour by hour, even minute by minute. It is change, then, that changes you and me. The *rapidity* of change and the *frequency* of change most influence our physical and mental health.

## Storm Defined

Simply stated, a storm is a change in the weather caused by the passage of large high and low pressure areas swirling and sweeping across a land mass or ocean (Mills, 57). What the public calls a storm is really the product of this condition: rising temperatures and "thunderhead" cloud formations, a calm period, then gusts of wind and pelting rain. Once this change has swept over us and away, we say that "the storm has passed." Actually, the air temperature has dropped, the barometer needle or mercury column registers a rise in atmospheric pressure, and the sky has started to clear. We have experienced change as it alternates, high to low and back to high atmospheric pressure, low to high and back to low atmospheric motion. We have experienced a storm in the technical sense, even without precipitation in the form of rain or frozen rain.

Storms vary in duration, some changes catching us unprepared by their abrupt appearance. Other changes may take place slowly, long enough to spoil the weekend, perhaps. Storms vary most markedly in degree of intensity, the inches of rain or snow that fall in an hour, which in turn is the product of wind speed. Some area populations accept their storms with what amounts to civic pride. The citizens of Boston, Massachusetts will quote mock (or real) weather predictions: "Sunny, followed by periods of rain, clearing by mid-afternoon, then thunder, hail, and snow. Tomorrow, cloudy and warmer." Kansans have a " 'Twarn't nothin' " attitude toward tornadoes, a storm experience many regional residents have endured. The Londoner seems to take a grim pleasure in three-day lows with accompanying fog. Australians, stoic through seasonal deluge and drought, know extreme changes of weather, and Texas "twisters" are the biggest and best, the stuff of folklore and legends. Storms in North America follow a rough pattern as they sweep across the continent. Wherever the movement of air masses is accompanied by change in temperature and pressure, the humans affected have experienced a storm, whether they got wet or not.

### North American Storm Patterns

The climate of the broad central basin of the continent of North America is quite different from the climates of the west and east coasts, each swept by the currents of the Pacific and Atlantic oceans. Two factors are involved that have human importance. The first is size. Over such a large, level land mass, the winters are colder and the summers hotter the farther the human dwells from a tempering ocean. Earth heats up faster and cools more quickly than does water. The second factor is horizontal space. The great central plains lie open to those frequent and sudden changes in atmospheric pressure called storms. The movement of great volumes of air is not checked by mountains or broad rivers hundreds of miles in length. Across large, flat land masses, anticyclones (high pressure systems) sweep from west to east. The direction of this movement makes the climate of New England cooler than that of southern Alaska, which enjoys the moderating effect of ocean currents moving up the Pacific coast.

Not only are the great plains of the central basin open to the west-to-east movement of anticyclones, but there is a sort of shallow trough or geological channel down which storms may flow, reaching the south central states, especially during the winter. Because of this channel, blizzards howl across the Oklahoma panhandle while Seattle, Washington records only a cool, cloudy spell. Anticyclones on the move east dip down south of the Great Lakes. Many plunge on down the valley of the Mississippi, their huge swirls churning up some very exciting weather in east Texas before moving on back up, roughly northeast, to make more snow in Buffalo, New York, or Bangor, Maine.

Cyclone air masses, turning around low pressure centers, are generally milder and tend to move more slowly. They pass across North America, beginning in Oregon and Washington, dipping only slightly in their slow flight over the great plains, then proceeding on east to fade out over the North Atlantic. While cyclones are usually less severe and less dramatic, they tend to duplicate the basic crude V-shape of North American weather. Storms begin in the west, slide across the country, then dip down, rise again and move northeast to complete the great V pattern. Low pressure and mild or high pressure and severe, these storms are changes powerful enough to affect human physical and mental health. What effects do storms have on us?

## How Weather Stimulates Cool-Climate Humans

We have been discussing natural climate and natural weather phenomena. Rapid and sharp changes brought about by storms roaming in the basic pattern of a huge V across the North American continent are natural changes. Precipitation may dampen human spirits as well as bodies, but rain need not fall for people to experience the quickening effect of a storm. Each such change generates vigor and physical restlessness, altering a number of basic body functions and resistance to disease. A storm, with or without snow or rain, is a strong stimulus to the entire human body and mind. At the same time, a storm endangers the human health it encourages (Mills, 57, 62).

Anthropologists, explorers, medical scientists, and zoologists have repeatedly observed that animal life is more active in cool climates than in the tropics. Humans born in temperate zones are demonstrably bigger—that is, both taller and heavier—than tropic zone humans. When humans are able to lose excess body heat, they can generate more heat to replace the loss. Available energy produced can be tapped in the form of work or vigorous play. The individual feels good, vital, and energetic. He tends to behave like it, full of noise and good humor and exhibiting an activity level he could not sustain in the hot, moist climate of the tropics.

A storm-stimulated human, reacting to the changes in his natural environment, is able to maintain good resistance to the sudden shifts of air temperature. He is adjusted to his own diurnal and circadian rhythms and to the alternating high and low pressures that sweep over the land he lives on. The cool-zone human, stimulated by his natural environment, is a stimulating fellow, at least to his geographical neighbors. With considerable exuberance, he has celebrated his own zest and praised his women for their vivacity, energy, and high-spirited charm. He has tended to fill his leisure hours with active games and to embellish his own life and surroundings with the fine and performing arts. He will stimulate himself, too, physically or mentally, "working up a sweat" in active exercise. He plays with the conditions of his environment, sliding on frozen rain, splashing in waters, running on the earth or riding over it. He responds to an environment that changes often enough to encourage all forms of activity.

Temperate man and his mate, together and apart, in small groups or large nations, have tended to be doers, inventive and restless makers and shakers. Like his weather, the cool-climate human manifests challenge and change. In the second chapter, we will consider the effects of weather on human moods and feelings. Here we will merely note in passing that temperate zone humans tend to be moody, given to quick anger as well as laughter, to sulks as easily as sport. The stimulated man and his mate are prone to all kinds of respiratory illnesses: colds, sinusitis, bronchitis, asthma, pneumonia, and tuberculosis, to name the most common. Since stimulation is a mental as well as a physical response, the cool male and his consort, often slowed or bed-ridden from disease, compensate by working or playing with extra vigor or energy "to make it up." This habit, partially caused by environment, partially a learned response inculcated by culture, takes the form of overwork, over-play, or overdoing which makes both males and females in temperate zones prey to cardiovascular diseases as well as respiratory diseases, as we shall see in Chapter 2.

## Scientific Studies of Weather Effects on Humans

The systematic examination of the effects of weather (as distinct from climate) on man seems to have begun nearly fifty years ago. Almost nobody these days has read a book called *Grundriss Einer Meteorobiologie des Menschens* and not a great many seemed to have examined the pages, not even Germans, who can read it with minimal effort and maximum understanding. This is a pity, since the author, named de Rudder, was among the first to try to help humans by explaining to them why they fell ill when they did. De Rudder's book is not easy to read, as the title may suggest, but he hammers out his thesis with typically temperate zone energy, providing a mass of statistics to prove his central point: when a storm front passes over a region (in his case, Germany), there is invariably a sharp rise in acute illness recorded by local physicians. Change triggers or contributes to disease.

De Rudder checked atmospheric pressures, air temperature readings, and admissions records kept by regional hospitals listing both date and presumed cause of admission. Sudden outbreaks of appendicitis, rheumatic fever, acute respiratory illnesses, what we might call "miniepidemics," occurred, according to de Rudder, just at the times when high or low fronts whirled across the area. Outside the range of local weather disturbance, de Rudder found hospital admissions to be normal, based on the experience of many years of operation. Although he did not claim that weather change caused disease, the German scientist was able to establish some evidence that weather disturbance and human disease were closely associated. It is understandable that his colleagues chose to disregard his work. Here was some Berliner, moaning in pain, while an intern checked for inflamed appendix. Where was *Herr Doktor* de Rudder? Examining the barometer!

*Meteorobiologie*, incidentally, is not German for "biometeorology," a Teutonic inversion, but rather expresses de Rudder's concept in cause-effect sequence: weather change coming before biological response to that change. This suggests an alternating pattern of health-illness-health more rigid than most medical scientists or meteorologists today would accept. Continuous monitoring of nat-

23

ural phenomena is now possible, due to revolutionary progress in electronic technology. No aspect of the universe now seems static to us. The constant is the constant of change. As weather is continuously becoming, so are the humans affected by it. We all are becoming better or worse in terms of physical well-being and, probably, in mental health as well. The aging processes alone are a slow degeneration of tissues, bones, and organs. Our solar system and our planet grow older every day. Climate and weather age, as well, although we seldom think of such huge environmental facts as subject to decay.

About a decade after the publication of de Rudder's pioneer study, two American medical scientists examined the interaction between weather and human health. Petersen's *The Patient and the Weather* confirmed the German doctor's findings. Smith sought to extend the range of research through an article in the *American Journal of Physiology*. Smith concentrated on a new area: mental health. Storm change as recorded in barometric pressures, he argued, appeared to have some cause-effect correspondence to disturbance in the human mind. When barometric pressures rise, the water balance in the human body goes to negative. Human body tissues respond to increased or lowered atmospheric pressure like a sponge; water is squeezed out and reabsorbed. Smith believed that water balance was related to those hard-to-explain but no less real feelings Americans had and still have. Not merely the "blahs," but odd, quirky fits of irrationality, cruelty, anger, and bad temper. Ancient physicians in Athens, Alexandria, and Rome were convinced that the human mind was sensitive to weather, climate, and natural environment. Storms high overhead seemed to churn and swirl deep human emotions, dreads, and instincts.

### The Moon and the Human Psyche

Three other American researchers, aware of moon-pull, tides, atmospheric pressure, and wind, patiently gathered information from over 1,500 weather stations that had each operated continuously for at least fifty years. They studied and published their findings: heavy rain fell in North America most often after the moon's full and new phases. Australians Adderley and Bowen found the same patterns held true "down under," confirming the research of Bradley, Woodbury, and Brier. The moon does affect the weather, which in turn causes physical responses that can be measured and mental reactions that are observable (Watson, 25).

Man has accepted himself as "moon-struck," probably long before the Romans endowed us with "lunatic" from their *lunaticus*. The original value of the word has been debased to the present "loony," or harmlessly insane, from the Latin sense of moon-influenced. Only since 1962 has there been certainty that weather itself is influenced as much by the moon as we believe ourselves can be. Scientific analysis often trails far behind our simply human hunches. The media common to a culture may transmit a superstition that research will clarify and confirm. Folk tales from both hemispheres and five continents, and dramatic works and novels of the Gothic school, perpetuated the belief that on nights when the moon is full the orthodoxy of nature eases and ghosts, werewolves, and vampires flit abroad at their hellish pleasures. Everybody knows Dracula. Hollywood has sustained many ancient terrors, often more effectively than it has been able to spook us with new horrors. Interesting facts established by biometeorologists around the world remind us of the bits of truth embedded in old myths and new movies.

When the moon is in its full phase, the recorded incidence of psychotically motivated crimes (arson, compulsive theft, symbolic and successful acts of self-destruction, atrocious assault and battery) tends to peak, even with heavy cloud cover over the locale of such antisocial acts. A study of 879 persons in the Philadelphia area correlated weather information and emergency admissions to city psychiatric wards. High barometric pressures were associated with persons seeking help for depression, while during low pressure days and nights admissions for intoxication were abnormally high. Fewer homicides occurred on sunny days than on cloudy days in 1973 (*New York Times*, May 10, 1974).

The Philadelphia study by Drs. Valentine, Ebert, Oakey, and Ernst included social conditions as well as environmental factors; crowded city streets tend to catch and hold a variety of pollutant materials at levels high enough to irritate both minds and bodies. Dutch research scientist S. W. Tromp summarized the apparent relationship between barometric pressures and suicide attempts in the Netherlands, and his evidence tends to confirm the study in Philadelphia, indicating "cluster days" of attempted self-slaughter.

Neurologist Leonard Ravitz has for years patiently measured the differences in electrical potential between the human head and chest. Utilizing extremely sensitive devices, he has been able to prove that the greatest differences between these head and chest measurements occur at full-moon phases. The greatest degree of difference he observed was in persons in mental institutions. In 1947 an early study indicated a worldwide tendency for death caused by tuberculosis to occur with greatest frequency on the seventh day prior to the full moon.

## The Difficulty of Interpreting Data

It is possible, of course, to make too much of scattered data. On the other hand, it should be noted that scientists of repute have neither reason nor inclination to seek information that would tend to confirm old wives' tales. Quite the reverse. Since World War II, approximately, there has been considerable reasoned interest in close studies of weather, climate, and man and his diseases. Pure data—that is, information correlating weather and human health—is hard to obtain. In a single generation, millions all over the earth have migrated from rural areas to big cities where social and cultural impacts too often combine with industrial and transportation pollutants creating quasitoxic environments. These days, the gigantic metropolitan areas are themselves localized weather-makers. The most common impact of the swollen city on the natural environment is that of the "heat-island," which tends to produce artificial rain, induced by masses of warm air rising from paved-over land masses encountering cool air above. In some urban centers, citizens go for days without a clear view of another powerful conditioner of weather and human health: the star that we call our sun (*Biometeorology*, Vol. 2, Part 2, 616).

## Sun Spots, Weather, and Health

The sun is an incandescent mass with a volume about a million times that of our earth. The core temperature has been estimated to be 13,000,000 degrees Centigrade. There, in a sort of super furnace, 4,000,000 tons of hydrogen burn up each second. Immense spouts of flame bubble and spew thousands of miles out from the surface of this star. The sun acts, too, like a continuous atom smasher, splitting off electrons and protons that pour away from the center as "solar wind" which touches and affects all the other planets in our modest little system.

The climate of the sun has been described just above, a continuous bubbling of surprisingly dense stuff. Given the fantastic rate at which hydrogen is consumed, the long average of conditions at the core and on the surface of this star is changing, but very slowly. The predicted life of the sun is reckoned in millions of years, even by the most pessimistic of observers.

The sun has its own weather, apparently caused by irregular

and especially violent activity near or on the surface, rather than by the impacts of any external force. Spots of molten matter about the size of our earth erupt or flare with such prodigious violence that various effects have been observed on our own planet. Sun-flare activity has been photographed by astronomers. Abrupt belches of energy appear to spread on the sun's surface, a form of rapid and violent change that corresponds to our definition of weather here on the earth.

Storm activity on the sun produces magnetic storms in our own atmosphere, "jamming" radio and television transmission. Most importantly, during periods of sun-flare, very large cyclones form over the oceans of the earth, while anticyclones appear over large land masses. Sun-flare activity tends to be associated with foul weather at sea and pleasant weather ashore. In theory, observed periods of abrupt change in the sun's weather should simplify weather predictions on our own planet. In fact, these storms on the surface of the star are highly irregular; only over long intervals can an apparent pattern be recorded. Interest began about 175 years ago, and many studies since have confirmed an eleven-year cycle of sun-flare activity corresponding to abnormal weather responses on our planet. Every eleven years, the larger lakes on our globe show a remarkable change in depth, the growth rings of trees are thicker, and glaciers fracture at a different rate, altering the number of icebergs broken off into Arctic waters. The subcontinent of India is visited by drought; every eleventh year additional tens of thousands perish of starvation there. Even a casual check of Burgundy wines will reveal that those judged to be great vintages come from grapes harvested eleven years apart (Watson, 29, 30).

Other studies suggest that the weather of the sun may affect the long average of conditions we call the climate of our earth. A long cycle of eighty to ninety years was noted by a German botanist interested in the annual bloom of a certain flower. Earthquake activity appears to rise for forty years, then decline to a low point. Over such extended time spans the rotation of the earth on its axis in annual progress through its orbit around the solar furnace apparently exposes all areas of our globe about equally to changes in the weather of the sun, causing changes in earth weather. As a final complication, the moon orbits the earth. A NASA document, "Initial Results of the IMP-1 Magnetic Field Experiment," provides data which indicates that the moon can deflect the speeding electrons and protons flung out from the sun as solar wind, thus causing some variation in the magnetic field of our planet.

## Body Weather

So long as sun weather creates or corresponds to the kinds of changes we have called weather here on earth, solar effects on human health must be considered indirect. Does the sun affect you and me in any sort of direct manner? Obviously so, since it generates and radiates both light and heat. The effects of solar radiation are so complex and have such significance that a more detailed discussion of light and human health is incorporated in chapter 3, and an extended analysis of heat effects on humans is contained in chapter 2. Here, we can note, in passing, some of the direct effects of the sun on human body chemistry.

### Solar Effects on Human Blood

Human blood, an amazingly complicated liquid that now constitutes a separate area of study by medical scientists, contains, among other substances, measurable amounts of albumin. Most humans know albumin best in the form of egg white. Until the late 1930s, the amount of albumin in human blood was believed to remain constant in men, but to vary in women with the menstrual cycle, which corresponds roughly to the lunar cycle of twenty-eight days. A Japanese researcher, noting what appeared to be a sudden rise in albumin level in both sexes, took blood samples and made a discovery that still bears his name: the Takata reaction. The results, an intriguing curve of daily variation among men, provided new information about the nature of blood and encouraged Takata to extend his studies.

Simply stated, the records of a decade showed that changes in the blood serum of Japanese males occurred most dramatically when significant sun flare activity altered the magnetic field of the earth. Additionally, the density of our planet's atmosphere was demonstrated to shield humans against excessive solar radiation. Takata's samples cover a period of about eleven years. The Japanese researcher, publishing in German, called the phenomenon he observed *kosmoterrestrischer Sympathismus* or "cosmoterrestrial sympathy," that is, an affinity or relationship in which what affects one thing (here, the sun) correspondingly affects another (man).

European researchers seem to have concentrated on another blood constituent, lymphocytes, small cells totaling no more than 25 percent of a normal human's white cell count. In year-long periods of solar bad weather, such as 1956–1957, the percentage of lymphocytes declined. February of 1956 was a remarkably explosive month on the surface of the sun. In Russia, hospital admissions for lymphocyte deficiencies were reported to have been twice the normal rate. Biometeorologists continue to observe the effects of the magnetic field disturbance caused by the sun on human blood. The proceedings of the Third International Biometeorological Congress, held in France in 1963, list no fewer than twenty-five papers reporting on solar radiation and the effects of it on the environment of the earth, with highly specific studies of magnetic field variations as contributing or sympathetic factors in the responses of plants, animals, and man. The recent abrupt and almost total disappearance of aerosol dispensers for hair conditioners, deodorants, and insect toxins dramatizes a contemporary awareness of man's dependence on the atmospheric shield controlling and limiting solar radiation.

Since human blood is pumped by the heart, and the statistics of mortality from all forms of coronary-vascular disease are truly terrifying, especially in North America, it is not so surprising to discover considerable research activity devoted to examining the impacts, direct and indirect, of the sun on the human heart and associated disfunctions and diseases. Scattered evidence now exists which suggests a relationship between sun flare and heart attack (myocardial infarction). The best-known work on this subject, *Correlations possibles entre l'incidence des infarctus du myocarde et l'augmentation des activités solaires et geomaneticques* by Poumailloux and Viart, is typically tentative. The relationship is "possible," not proved. The thesis the French physicians advance is that solar activity may promote the formation of blood clots in predisposed humans. No one claims that sun flare causes heart attack. Many of the studies made, seeking to provide better information on the relationship between man and the sun of his planetary system, concentrate on the effects of heat radiation, solar heating of environmental air, and the metabolic stress of heat loss during warm weather periods. More questions have been asked than answers found. Even some evidence seems contradictory. Why, if sun flares possibly induce blood clotting, do they seem to correlate with hemorrhage in the lungs of tuberculosis victims?

It seems fair to state, in summary of this rather generalized overview of climate, weather, and human health, that humans have been quite aware of climatic and weather stimulation and stress for thousands of years. Some very early observations have been confirmed, but much has been discarded as simply untrue or random evidence, thanks to increasing interest in life reactions to environment and more sophisticated instruments and methods of measurement. It is also occasionally puzzling to read the results of medical research tending to ignore or disregard the effects of natural environmental conditions upon human well-being. On this continent the tendency has been to treat disease through drug therapy. Put the control or the cure in a pill or a needle. There is good reason for this, to be sure. Results can be estimated with fair accuracy and dangerous guesswork reduced if not eliminated. The interior space of the incredibly intricate human body, when measured by trillions of highly specialized cells, is really vast, but much smaller than the immensity of cosmic space and forces. The body weather of the individual is, proportionately at least, easier and less expensive to manage than is the weather of our environment, with which we exist in sympathetic and still mysterious association. The doctor and the patient himself can do something about the weather *inside* the human body, creating or checking the storms of disfunction or disease. Human blood pressure can be modified for millions by drugs and diet therapy. Atmospheric pressure, on the other hand, cannot be controlled for humans, except for those very few that briefly dwell in the depths of the sea or in the cold vastness of airless space. In point of fact, humans do not live in bathyspheres or capsules and never will. It is known that, to varying degrees, human attempts to control and modify climate and weather, replacing the natural with the artificial, has not been an unalloyed good. For every step along the road of Progress, we have been obliged to pay a sometimes invisible or unnoticed price. Efforts to increase convenience and comfort have caused new effects on human physical and mental health. The section that follows will seek to make the reader more aware of artificial climate and weather as health conditioners.

## ARTIFICIAL CLIMATE, CONDITIONED WEATHER, AND MODERN MAN

Assume a contemporary Scot, an executive for Byrnam Wood Products & Dunsinane Distributors, Ltd., and dress him in a synthetic fiber three-piece double-knit business suit instead of chain-link battle dress and steel helmet. He does not ramble on a misty moor, but strolls into a modern office building. Market reports from the London exchange indicate a future filled with promise and peril. Like Shakespeare's creation, our modern Macbeth has reason to exclaim, "So foul and fair a day I have not seen."

Can he be talking of the weather, still? How is this possible? His skyscraper office offers temperate-zone conditions at all times.

Elaborate equipment in the basement and on the roof works continuously to maintain a constant temperature, regardless of external conditions. Inside, it is always sixty-five degrees Fahrenheit. Glass walls, tinted to reduce the glare of solar radiation and to retard the passage of both ultraviolet and infrared rays, serve to protect him from disturbing draughts and distracting chill. Overhead, acoustical tile ceilings muffle office noises and naturally inert gases glow in fluorescent lighting tubes that totally control the illumination of all surfaces beneath. Filters trap and reduce the levels of particulates in the air he breathes, neutralizing the potential dangers of minute bits of dust, fly ash, sulphur dioxide, and hydrocarbons surely more measurably toxic than the contents of any witches' cauldron.

Since moving with his wife to Glamis Tower, a high-rise apartment, our modern Macbeth is never subject to the inconvenience or discomfort experienced by his forebears. Central heat, conditioned air, electric light, and moisture control are all at his fingertips. Why, his home is a model of modern living, so conducive to good health that his lady has ceased to walk in her sleep, although perhaps the ready availability of certain spot removers and synthetic cleansers have combined to ease her mind. All is so evidently fair that a surly suggestion that it could be anything less than splendid in all ways is "foul," indeed. A peril to the health? Ridiculous!

Let us grant, at once and without quibble, that modern man employed in a contemporary technologically advanced nation or region enjoys, in his home at least, comforts no monarch of the past could ever purchase or cause to be created. The very bed he sleeps in is engineered for ease, and hundreds of mechanical horses transport him in a day farther than a royal progress could creep in a week. Ancient kings, as their chroniclers inform us, died as readily as any slave, although with considerably more drama. An Egyptian pharaoh may have eased an agony with opium, but modern Egyptians can purchase aspirin in exchange for only a few moments of their labor, converted into cash. There can be no question that when existence is measured in innersprings, miles per hour, or fast, safe relief from simple distress, contemporary man enjoys a princely lifestyle that the long-dead would envy.

Until the advance of technology—specifically, the ability to control and make use of new power sources—what the king could buy that his subjects could not was largely decoration and distraction. The royal family could shiver within gorgeous apartments. Dressed in velvets, lace, and jewels, they could look at and listen to various court entertainments. They ate the same approximate diet as their own servants, with utensils of silver or gold. In all other aspects, each one a significant contributing factor to human health, the king shared the same environment with the commoner. When it came to the weather and the climate, all men were equal.

## The Urban Microclimate

Now contemporary technology has created what British biometeorologist M. Parry may have been the first to term "microclimates" (*Biometeorology*, Vol. 2, Part 2, 623). A microclimate is normally found in describable state within an urban area. Using our original definition of climate as the long average of affecting environmental conditions, it should not be hard to understand that our modern Macbeth dwells in two such microclimatic areas, hypothetically separated by only a short distance, easily traversed in his air-conditioned and heated automobile, inside which he shuttles twice daily from his domestic microclimate to his executive microclimate. Assuming that his apartment is located within the same city where he works, our contemporary Scot may quit the urban heat-island only on his holidays and occasional weekends. Except for these excursions, the urban citizen anywhere exists within one or two microclimates that minimize his exposure to natural sunlight, solar-heated air, the cooling effect of moving air masses, and regional precipitation. Urban dwellers now measure their contacts with what used to be called "fresh air" by exposure-minutes. An objection that certain workers (traffic police and construction workers come first to mind) spend their working hours outdoors must be countered by the observation that the concrete canyons of a modern city typically bear no measurable resemblance to what could be termed a natural environment. Such workers are more rightly considered to be exposed to the fullest impacts of heat-island climate and weather, regardless of actual geographic location. They are simply not so totally enclosed.

Since modern man everywhere has increasingly shown his desire to migrate from rural to urban areas, thus reversing the amount of time he exposes himself to natural conditions and rhythms as against the artificial, a brief summary of the basic microclimate affecting his health may be in order.

### The Heat-Island

While it is unreasonable to blame individuals for the health-affecting environment of the modern city, it is possible to note that several men developed the processes now combined to build what critic Lewis Mumford calls the tyrannopolis: the gathering of all races and nationalities in an area engineered to such density of humans per square foot that all aspects of life are subject not to human will but to the perpetual malfunctioning of the city itself. Macadam perfected a type of durable paving compounded of asphalt that can be poured, spread, and rolled. Eiffel erected bolted skeletons greater in vertical dimension than in the horizontal space they occupied. Louis Sullivan wrapped steel girders in a concrete envelope. Ford mass-produced the automobile. For all practical purposes, the tyrannopolis was born about fifty years ago. We have seen that pure responses, unconditioned by social and cultural factors, are no longer easy to assay and we shall make no serious attempt to consider, beyond predeclared limits, the health effects of vehicle congestion, human overcrowding, accident hazards, and dwindling human and financial resources directed to maintain health. It must remain a hope, for the most part, that the implications of admittedly and deliberately limited discourse will urge the reader to reflect on the war urban man is losing to tyrannopolis. To the degree that M. Parry makes possible, let us here contemplate the city as the most frequently encountered microclimate:

> The urban structure, essentially one of horizontal and vertical surfaces of brick, stone and concrete, has a relatively low albedo [fractional electromagnetic reflection from a surface], and a large heat capacity so that it absorbs strongly the incoming solar radiation of the day, stores much of its heat and releases it slowly during the evening and night, while the moist green vegetation-clad countryside not only absorbs less solar energy but it must expend some of it on the evaporation of moisture and use scme of it chemically in photosynthesis. Today it is recognized also that urban smoke haze may well deplete incoming radiation thus possibly reducing day-time temperatures in the town below those of the surrounding country, but the same factor is even more effective at night, by blanketing the town and preventing the radiative heat loss which proceeds unchecked in rural areas. To these may be added the heat loss from buildings, mainly during the heating season, and that liberated by the metabolism of a concentrated population and from the exhausts of motor vehicles.

The central concept here is that of solar energy and heat, a conversion process Parry accurately names as metabolism. (The single qualification of consequence to this otherwise admirable definition would be that the microclimate of the heat-island is affected by heat loss from buildings year-round, because of the widespread use of air conditioning equipment which pumps uncalculated amounts of hot air and tons of water vapor into the surrounding atmosphere.) With the basic concept—metabolism—before us as the prime fact of climate and weather, let us leave our imaginary modern Macbeth poised to begin his workday inside a modern microclimate and consider man as a fueled machine, an ambulating metabolic apparatus.

From the misted dawn of prehistory to the smoggy dusk of today, man's most consistent and successful efforts at controlling his climate and his weather have been directed at modification of air temperature. What man has worked with outside his body is what works inside his frame: the process we call combustion.

### The Human Body as Internal Combustion Engine

In some regions, humans exist at levels barely above that of self-propelled vegetables, as they have lived for centuries. Temperate zone humans are inclined to view tropical peoples as "lazy"; yet one of the most primitive human subgroups was discovered by Charles Darwin near the tip of South America, a region distinguished by a cold climate. The near-bestial people Darwin met were exceptional, truly primitive compared to either Eskimos or Australian aborigines, each inhabiting extreme climates and enjoying good success with sufficient leisure and inclination to produce sophisticated works of art. Tierra del Fuego, on the other hand, posed problems of combustion that the indigenous tribe Darwin observed had been unable to solve, except internally, that is, by eating.

We have indicated above that in cooler zones, humans are stimulated, stimulating, and stressful creatures, restless, seemingly urged by environment and culture to be busy at work and play. Cool-climate humans often die, as one of their poets noted with compassion, "of a rage to live." The most important factor in determining the *level* (another long average of many conditions) at which a population may exist is the energy they find available for their use and misuse. This energy for growth, thought, and action is derived solely from the internal combustion of their foods, modified by the climatic impact of solar radiation. Since the sun-warmed seasons affect plant and animal life, the range and variety of available food depends, naturally enough, on the weather.

Human beings are incredibly complex, but not especially efficient machines, when considered exclusively as internal combustion engines. Like the machines we have invented, we waste much of our fuel. Other animal species convert food by combustion to usable energy at a higher rate of efficiency (the horse and the dog, for examples). Humans turn fuel to power at about the same efficiency rate as an old-fashioned noncondensing steam engine during weather periods dominated by low atmospheric pressure. Tropical humans function at about that low rate for a lifetime. Temperate humans or all persons in weather conditioned by high atmospheric pressure operate at about the rate of efficiency of a Model A Ford automobile.

## Cooling and Heating Mechanisms of the Human Body

The great amounts of waste heat that humans generate in the process of converting food fuels to energy has necessitated an adequate and delicately balanced cooling mechanism. An automobile engine, typically idle most of the time, needs to warm up. Man's internal combustion system, which never shuts off, needs to be cooled. With a normal level of temperature hovering at 98.6 degrees Fahrenheit, the human body undergoes severe disturbance of physical and mental functions if that internal temperature varies by as much as a single degree. Even a rise of .5 degree on the Fahrenheit scale has mildly disruptive consequences. This being so, it is probable that prehistoric man learned to cool his naked body by immersion in water or mud before he discovered he could trap his own excess body heat with a layer of animal skins. Then, many tens of thousands of years later, he taught himself and his heirs the knack of external combustion, the deliberate use of fire to modify the air temperature of his living quarters.

Under typical conditions in a cool climate, the nerve-controlled blood supply to the skin capillaries and sweat glands is adequate to regulate and to make possible the loss of excess body heat produced by the food-converting process. However, this system of automatic self-cooling is effective for only short intervals and serves to lower body temperature only slightly. Conversely, if the surrounding air temperature is too cool for too long (a matter of only a few moments), our body weather changes and we experience *hyperpyrexia*. We "feel chilly." If the cool condition persists, our internal combustion system steps up to counter a rapid and enduring heat loss. Under normal conditions, nude, unsheltered humans have little usable excess energy with which to create a culture. So long as we are obliged to consume the energy derived from food in self-cooling or self-heating, we tend to remain much as we were. Probably, the combination of accident and memory enabled very early man to make the first gestures toward those willed patterns of activity anthropologists call "culture."

### Heat, Cold, and Oxygen Consumption

When external temperature falls, oxygen intake rises. Just as wood or fossil fuels require oxygen to burn, so we must have the life-sustaining gas to burn the stuff we have eaten or have stored in our body cells. This response to cool air is almost immediate. The decrease in temperature is passed from nerve endings to the brain and back to the muscles. We chafe our chilled fingers together, swing our arms, or jump up and down "to get the blood moving." This use of the muscles very swiftly depletes the energy already stored in the tissues. More oxygen is needed to convert this "banked" energy into use-energy. We do not merely inhale automatically; we gasp deliberately, pulling the oxygen into our lungs. Heartbeat rate increases and our blood moves, pouring through the lungs, picking up free oxygen and rushing it to the muscle tissues, and carrying off waste products to be vented through our complex exhaust systems.

Like other animals, humans can and do learn to tolerate different temperature levels, but it is a response to conditioning. Laboratory animals raised in rooms kept cooler than normal for their species can then be shifted to another area, still cooler, and withstand chilling much better than the same species not preconditioned. A few animal species store glycogen, a kind of antifreeze secretion. Humans do not. Unable to adapt so readily to the conditions of existence, man alters the conditions so he may exist more comfortably. If the slow passage of the seasons may be said to have a human purpose (an assumption only a pious fundamentalist would make), then each is a conditioner for the succeeding season. Modern man, dweller in microclimates, has all but lost awareness of the seasons. Historically, the records show that seventeenth-century immigrants to the North American continent died by the dozens in Massachusetts settlements, while a few miles away, the Algonquin Indians (who wore noticeably less clothing summer and winter) survived.

In more recent decades, medical scientists quibbled over the scattered evidence gathered from testing of human heat-production levels, trying to prove, one way or the other, that seasonal changes in human metabolism did or did not occur. At length, it was established beyond question that a definite and fairly regular decline in consumption of oxygen took place when mean air temperature level rose, one of those measurable inverse relationships that so delight the scientific mind. Temperature down, oxygen use up and vice versa. When Dr. Knunde reported in the early 1930s that her own metabolism during the first four days of her menstrual cycles averaged 9 percent lower in oxygen consumption in the summer than in the winter and when Dr. Kakagawa was able to prove that the children he observed grew at different rates at different seasons, much of the scientific world seems to have said, "Uh-huh," shrugged its white-coated shoulders, and gone about its business. After all, women were physical oddities prone to easy tears and Japanese kids looked so different it was hardly surprising that they grew in some peculiar local fashion (Mills, 10).

Yet the fact that oxygen consumption varies with the seasons and that the human use of this combustion-supporting gas is always controlled by external mean air temperature and resulting ease or difficulty of heat loss was and is an important discovery. Since seasonal fluctuations in temperature are widest in temperate climates, it is in these cool, changeable zones where the most basic bodily processes are most affected by changes in the weather. Humans are extremely sensitive to environmental factors affecting heat loss. Cool-climate man, through his very activity in response to natural stimulation, has altered his surroundings more than has tropical man. In seeking artificial means of increasing his own convenience, efficiency, and comfort, temperate man has damaged his own environment, creating microclimates never before experienced and poisoning the air he, especially, has need of to an unprecedented degree. Given some choice in the matter, North Americans have rather conspicuously preferred to cool the air rather than make it clean.

### Heat and Human Health

When air temperature rises, making loss of body heat difficult, animal growth in all species slows down and sexual maturity is delayed. When grown to adults, animals of the tropic zones tend to be lean and light in ratio of weight to height. Since fertility is late, animal groups in the tropics typically have a low birth rate, experiencing some difficulty in conception, with stillbirth quite common. While animals existing in energy-depressing, hot, moist climates exhibit only moderate physical and mental activity, they seldom die in the middle years, tend to look younger longer, and generally remain healthy despite old age. On the other hand, tropical animals chill easily and have little resistance to infections. Naturally, we include man as a tropic-zone animal.

As mean air temperatures cool, permitting easy loss of body heat, all animal growth tends to be rapid, with the young maturing quickly and body weight, height, and muscle mass combining in robust, round forms. Fertility is typically early and easy. Infants are born in large numbers; stillbirth and infant mortality rates are low. As we have seen, temperate-zone animals are vital and energetic creatures, able to tolerate variable conditions of weather and to resist infection. More regularly stimulated and therefore more highly stressed, temperate-zone animals tend to suffer systemic breakdowns leading to death in middle age or even youth. Overall, temperate zone animals tend to live shorter lives than their tropical counterparts (Mills, 12). Again, this is as true of men as it is of mice.

Heat loss is typically effected by radiation, conduction, or convection. Evaporation, an emergency response, usually takes care of the rest. The radiation of heat directly from the skin surface to the air is the easiest and fastest method and can be the only one needed to maintain normal internal body temperature in man. The rate of heat loss is more important to human well-being than the method. Once this fact was known, technological skills were employed to maintain optimum temperatures through artificial means. Climate control and weather conditioning is concerned with radiation: external heat is transported and radiated into the air within which humans live, work, and rest, or the surrounding air is chilled to make body heat radiated from humans easily dissipated. These short-term modifications of climate and weather have become living habits to the degree that citizens of technologically advanced states now notice the artificial only when it is absent. Power failures or "brown-outs" dramatize how much we have accepted our own dependency on the artificial.

### Acclimatization

Yet man, like other animals, is quite adaptable to long-term climatic change. When human families migrate from hot climates to cooler zones, the first-generation offspring exhibit the characteristics of all young born into and raised in temperate zones; size and weight to height ratios change to conform to the young of parents living in cool-climate conditions for many generations. Acclimatization for adults seems to take several years. The chemistry of the blood undergoes changes not yet perfectly known, although humans adapted to heat do have "thinner" blood.

The old saying "It's not the heat; it's the humidity!" appears to be quite valid. An Australian transferred from Sydney to Sumatra will not experience great change in mean air temperature, but Sydney is dry heat and Sumatra is moisture-laden heat. In a year or so, he feels nothing special about humidity that originally seemed enervating, even exhausting. Shipped home, but this time to Perth, where the climate is comparable to that of San Francisco, the Australian will experience discomfort from chill, although the humidity may be about the same as in Sumatra. Persons who have grown acclimated to tropical humidity can endure only a few degrees drop in air temperature. The Australian in question here will shiver at readings still well above comfort levels of temperate zones. Effectively tropicalized, he will have lost some of his capacity to resist infection and may well contract the all-too-common cold. His body is responding to changes in weather and climate, alterations in the degree of stimulation experienced.

### Index of Climate Stimulation

By a relatively simple system of correlating temperature readings with some correcting factors that reduce statistical variables, an index of climate stimulation was arrived at nearly forty years ago (Mills, 86-88). Consider the following selection:

| Station | Index of Stimulation |
|---|---|
| Minneapolis | 18.5 |
| San Francisco | 14.6 |
| Charleston, S.C. | 13.4 |
| Houston | 12.4 |
| | |
| Panama City | 3.0 |
| Honolulu | 2.9 |
| Bombay | 2.3 |
| Entebbe (Uganda) | 1.3 |

Obviously, a human moving from Bombay to Minneapolis would experience such an increase in stimulation that he might suffer severe stress, metabolic collapse, and infectious or degenerative disease. The Texan traveling from Houston to Panama City would suffer correspondingly from the change in climate and weather. He would be more susceptible to the diseases common to the tropics than a native Panamanian. The history of nineteenth-century colonial and commercial expansion is full of examples where these facts were ignored. Transplanted humans suffered and died by the tens of thousands, before their first-generation offspring were born. The index above is based on natural data, taken long enough ago to be no longer accurate. The heat-island effect of Minneapolis-St. Paul caused by massive building in recent decades has no doubt caused a drop in its index rating, while Honolulu's almost total air conditioning constitutes its new microclimate.

What is considered "ideal" or at least optimum as stimulation expressed numerically? About 14.5, or the climate of San Francisco.

### Central Heating

Improving systems of heating enclosed air has utilized much human inventiveness and millions in resources across the centuries. The cool and stormy continent of North America, combined with abundant natural fuels, spurred migrants to control the temperature of their dwellings so as to produce an energy surplus which they could expend in other achievements. Control over the numbing and exhausting effects of winter through central heating is not without health effects. Typically, North American homes and work spaces tend to be both too hot and too dry. Many experience dessication of the mucous membranes of the nose or mouth, throat irritation caused by drying, loss of appetite, dulling headache, and the dimly perceived but no less discomforting sensation of suffocation.

As desirable temperate areas were settled and exploited, North Americans turned to fertile subtropical and tropical zones, centers of easy, abundant growth of foodstuffs and useful fibers. Having solved by inventiveness in concert with resources the problem of moderating cold weather, man progressed more slowly with the difficult task of modifying the depressing effects of too much heat and too much moisture. It has proved both easier and healthier to combat winter chill than to cool summer heat.

### Air Conditioning

Modern thermal engineers and appliance manufacturers have made great progress in enabling people to create and maintain almost any sort of climate desired, provided it is artificial. The air-conditioning industry began without much basic information about body reactions to abrupt temperature change, human metabolism, and disease. Only approximates of comfort guided the development of air-cooling equipment. Engineers schemed to make this apparatus less bulky, cheaper to build, easier to install and maintain, and more efficient, all attributes that would increase sales, not human health. Medical scientists and physiologists were rather slow in bringing their methods of investigation and control to bear on the new problems created inadvertently by the drive to solve an old problem of human comfort. Recently—that is, within the past two decades—a new cooperation has developed between biologists and climate engineers. The general public, however, remains innocent.

The average purchaser simply installs a unit and turns it on, just as his parents did with the oil furnace and the electric light bulb. Humans have always craved comfort and convenience. In the Western democracies at least, the right to consume is limited only by available net income, and most persons exercise this right without much regard for health consequences. Yet it is a truism that any good carried to excess can become bad.

As mentioned earlier, it is the rate of heat loss that determines the tempo and rhythms of human energy levels and active achievements. Too little heat loss suppresses human combustion, reducing energy excess. Too great heat loss leads to metabolic exhaustion and sharply decreased vitality. If the rate is optimum, then the human enjoys maximum well-being, both sensed and actual. The problem is maintaining heat loss at the optimum level, complicated by the fact that few humans agree on the standard they should share. Once it was discovered that factory and office work efficiency could be boosted in the summer months by about 30 percent more than that observed when working-space temperatures rose about the level comfortable to all, then group productivity rather than the comfort of individuals controlled the hand that controlled the switch.

### Health Hazards of Ministorms

Dangerous or unhealthy working conditions are a legitimate grievance for both blue- and white-collar employees. Yet spotwelders, supermarket clerks, and stenographers seem not to believe they should control the air temperature conditions under which they work. Temperature control is an odd form of totalitarian manipulation, and few employees (or family members) feel free to object to its abuse. Instead, we surrender ourselves to a series of microclimatic ministorms over a full quarter of the year. In our interior spaces, we have agreed to abolish the summer season. We don sweaters to shop in frigid stores and markets, often as much as twenty-five degrees cooler than the air outside. We do not acclimatize our bodies through natural responses to a natural environment. We overstimulate and overstress our systems through the overuse of air conditioning to increase employee efficiency.

### The Summer Cold

Like alcoholism, the common cold is extremely democratic and ranks as a major cause of worker/student absenteeism. Since air conditioning has become commonplace, so has the "out of season" cold. For untold hundreds of thousands, the summer has become a season of sneezes, postnasal drip, and sore throat, as well as sunburn. A factory or office worker, cooled like a slaughterhouse carcass for eight hours each day, soon does not feel that he is comfortable outside this chilled microclimate. As he passes from home to street to place of labor and back, he subjects himself to a half-dozen ministorms daily. The protective mucous linings that shield delicate membranes of nose and throat are repeatedly chilled and heated. The glands pump extra fluids, slow down, and are triggered to overwork again. The tops of the lungs regularly experience abrupt twenty- to thirty-degree differences in air temperature, while the metabolism is shocked by fluctuations in humidity of 200 percent. Nonsmokers stressed by these conditions hack away like addicts. The overstimulated worker drags himself home, exhausted by experiencing January in July, kisses a spouse or friend, and both come down with "colds" in midsummer.

Despite absenteeism, complaints, and scattered warnings, most industrial or commercial air conditioning units are set to create air temperatures of 70 degrees Fahrenheit. In June, this may not be too far from the mean daily temperature, although the sensitive will feel the early effects of the microclimate. By early August, however, such a setting is much too cold, harmful chilling is commonplace, and the rate of infectious disease mounts sharply. (The taxpayer-promoted scheme of year-round schooling, designed to make more efficient use of facilities idle during the summer season, fails to consider the undesirable impact upon children experiencing not a single climate to which their bodies have gradually adjusted but two, with real adjustment to either made impossible by alternation.)

The same setting is typical of artificial environments in North America during the winter months as well. In fact, thermostatic control can moderate interior temperatures in offices, schools, apartments, and private homes year-round, gradually conditioning resident bodies to accept this arbitrary setting as the acceptable norm. There seems to be no more indication that seventy degrees warmth is good for you in the winter than seventy degrees of chill is health-promoting in the summer. Quite the contrary, for what has been abandoned is *optimum change*, from season to season—the slow, almost imperceptible acclimatization to temperate zone stimulation and relaxation our bodies are designed to enjoy.

Under natural conditions (these days, that is a state experienced only outdoors) humans individually control the loss of excess body heat by wearing more or less clothing in response to the surrounding air temperature across the slow span of the seasons. Nude, we radiate heat constantly, in straight rays moving close to the speed of light until they strike any object that can absorb them and thus be warmed, in turn, by the heat we have thrown off. At the same time, our bodies are generally subjected to solar radiation, either direct or filtered through cloud cover. We are then objects absorbing warmth from the sun. In both instances, molecular motion of the air that surrounds us is involved. In contact with our skin, the warmed air increases in temperature, then physically moves away, the conduction-convection process. Clothing slows this process by intervening layers of natural or artificial fabric. Cottons, linens, and light fibers woven with a loose or open mesh conduct body heat to the air more quickly and, therefore, more easily. Winter woolens, furs, and tight acrylic fabrics make excellent insulation, slowing the loss of heat by radiation and conduction-convection.

The actual rate of heat loss is determined by the difference between how hot we are and the temperature of the surrounding air. Capillaries permit maximum access of the blood to the skin surface. Air motion, a breeze sliding over the exposed skin, removes the closest layer of heated air, replacing it with a cooler layer. Thus, the rate remains constant or may increase slightly with the wind speed in miles per hour. When this system does not work fast enough, we sweat.

As the salty water exuded from the sweat glands pours onto the skin, it vaporizes in contact with the already heated skin surface. Sweating is a remarkably effective safety system protecting you against overheating and sun stroke. The big "if" about sweating is not the brand name of the deodorant you choose, but the degree that the air around you is already water-saturated. The lower the humidity, the more rapidly human sweat can evaporate.

### How Air Conditioning Affects Human Ailments

Air conditioning both chills air and lowers its moisture within an enclosed space. In general, dry air is bad for humans. The humidity level should only be low enough to permit sweat vaporization as needed, itself a human variable. Physical labor or energetic play will cause your personal radiator to boil over, but desk work or study won't. Slowly but steadily, the body adjusts to external environment—or can, given the chance. Work or play can be accomplished in August, with no sweat, whereas the same amount of activity in June would have left you drenched in perspiration.

An arbitrary and automatic setting of seventy degrees, winter and summer, regardless of activity level, is senseless as well as health-threatening. Microclimate conditions should be adjusted to permit body heat loss to be accomplished with ease just under the point of active sweating. At present, most of us rarely enjoy optimum microclimatic conditions. Almost always, we are stressed by excessive chilling of the air. Air-motion control is difficult, even in enclosed spaces. The typical home air conditioning system does not attempt to control the motion of air. Only in old-fashioned stores and restaurants are we likely to feel the benign effects of big, ceiling-mounted fans. Aging newspaper reporters sometimes recall the corner saloons with smaller fans blowing beery breezes over cakes of ice set in wash tubs. Uncontrolled air motion permits stratification with cooler layers near the floor and warmer layers pushed above. Stratification may cause mild discomfort through localized chilling, through draughts, or the peculiar sensation of being exposed to several air temperatures at once.

Our modern microclimates are created with one eye fixed firmly on cost. Obviously, if walls, floors, and ceiling were simultaneously cooled, the human heat radiated to these flat surfaces could be absorbed in massive amounts. But the cost of cooling a wall is many times greater than fabricating a miniature refrigeration mechanism with intake and exhaust fans, which is all an air conditioning unit really is. While it is true that some work and living spaces in North America have radiant heating systems, with pipes or conduits embedded in concrete floor slabs, no comparable system of radiant cooling exists outside specialized research or laboratory facilities.

Modern fiberglass insulation approximates and even exceeds the capacity of solid stone or adobe walls, although typically the modern home is so insulated only in the attic floor or roof. Here again, comfort and cost factors collide. Since hot air rises, the effectiveness of fiberglass insulation is limited to holding heat generated by the home furnace inside the house as a sort of lid. The glass walls of contemporary structures, unless they are doubled with an air space between (a doubled cost), permit the easy exchange of heat and cold at all seasons. Modern office buildings are designed more for aesthetic impact than human comfort, and some of our contemporary glass towers might well be considered to constitute health hazards, both because of what happens to people working and living inside them and accidents inflicted on passers-by below when the flat panels of glass explode from pressure and wind shifts or shatter from too rapid expansion and contraction. Humans acclimatize more readily than habitations.

It seems fair to say that, over all, a considerable number of diseases and disturbed metabolic functions can be influenced for the better by controlled climate and weather. Air conditioning units at work or in the home, if regulated according to need rather than simply set once and thereafter tolerated, can be used as legitimate therapy or preventive medicine. Misused, the same equipment can help create or worsen health situations it might prevent or improve. Moreover, climatic therapy permits prompt and sure benefits for some diseases in which alternate forms of treatment are difficult, expensive, or unpredictable.

What is now known that was not understood a few decades ago is that the standard modern habit of existing within one or more artificial microclimates in defiance of seasonal change and varying bodily needs tends to combine many factors of body weather harmful to human physical and mental well-being. Artificial heating and chilling, artificial illumination, artificial methods of food processing and storage, lack of physical exercise on a regular basis, and excessive and valueless stimulation of the senses have combined to make too many North Americans fat and feeble, exactly the opposite of how we would like to be, as individuals, families, and groups. We cannot blame that sad condition on the weather, since we have made it, to a large degree. Thus aware, we can consider some specific therapeutic possibilities and potential threats created by our new ability to manufacture climate and weather.

Since adjustment to new climatic conditions seems to take many months, it is fair to say that the climate to which we are accustomed is carried with us when we migrate, make a long visit, and return. Many of the most common forms of infection in temperate regions appear to be conditioned by sudden storm changes, that is, by atmospheric factors. Few persons afflicted with chronic respiratory troubles can afford permanent migration from New England or the northern Midwest to Arizona. A better move might be west to the San Francisco Bay area, where greater atmospheric calm combines with health-stimulating cool temperatures.

No one suffering from chronic respiratory illness should move to lowland regions of subtropical warmth and high humidity. Persistent bronchitis in Minneapolis or Montreal will not vanish in Miami. However, at an elevation such as that of New Mexico, bronchial attacks should lessen while vitality and resistance stabilize at a relatively high level.

There is no air conditioning system that manufactures New Mexico's climate. In fact, the excess stimulation of an air conditioner extended into the summer months may actually lower resistance to infection and could prove worse than no relief from excess heat at all. A natural climate, if not completely health-supporting, offers chances of reduced harm compared to over- or misuse of artificial climate controls. If used, adjust home air conditioning no more than ten degrees cooler than exterior air temperatures on warm days. Avoid interior winter season heat above seventy degrees. Set the home thermostat in the mid-sixties. Help your body acclimatize by regular, moderate outdoor exercise.

In diseases attributed in whole or in part to malfunctioning metabolism, the possibilities of therapy through climate control should be discussed with the family physician. Many metabolic disfunctions affect cardiac capacity, the ability of the heart muscle to accomplish its needed work. In general, the goal should be to avoid stress, the sort of stimulation that leads to physical exhaustion and requires the body to labor hard in order to maintain healthful heat loss. Historically, therapy has included advice to abandon strenuous physical labor and recreation, to change employment if it involves competition with calendars and clocks, and to vacation in or move to a warmer climate.

Artificial weather control can help to the degree that a home conditioning unit will serve to make body heat loss easier. This may be especially beneficial at night, when rest permits many body systems to repair damage. Surrounded by cool air, the cardiac patient under care of a physician and obedient to the doctor's instructions will be helped to avoid heart strain. Less energy and effort will be expended in cooling the body; the heart will not be obliged to work at dangerous levels. Total inactivity is seldom suggested by doctors treating persons with metabolic disfunctions. Controlled or limited activity may be advised while the total rehabilitation program is monitored. Eased sleep and comfortable days, with moderation in all activities, is the best body weather for metabolic problems.

Rheumatic infections, as well as those which strike the respiratory system, seem to be associated with sudden, sharp weather change within a generally stimulating climate. Rheumatic infections appear often as secondary to, and possibly proceeding from, respiratory illness. The incidence of both jumps during the stormy winter season in a temperate zone. The standard drug therapy is controlled dosage with penicillin, shown to be very effective in combat with rheumatic fever, that insidious crippler of young hearts.

In modern microclimates, body chilling has become a summer threat as well as a winter worry. Artificial climate control offers only partial therapy for rheumatic diseases that typically damage the valves of the human heart. Constant temperatures—or at least a narrow range, plus low humidity—will allow the heart to work with minimized strain. Migration, to be effective, must be permanent and, ideally, to areas above 5,000 feet. A number of infections can enter a dormant phase, but are capable of resurgence if the sufferer is exposed to northern cold accompanied by sudden atmospheric changes.

The health benefits of the American Southwest—Arizona and New Mexico, especially—are not propaganda distributed by chambers of commerce and travel agents. Many tens of thousands of North Americans have discovered that life at altitudes 5,000 feet above sea level is, indeed, a health-sustaining "high." Overall, the degree to which artificial climates can simulate a naturally supporting environment is limited. No home, school, or office air conditioning unit manipulates atmospheric pressure. Yet the experience of those persons unable or unwilling to migrate does indicate that real benefits can be obtained by persons already suffering from impaired heart functions.

Some preventive benefits, too, can accrue to persons aware of a family history of congestive heart failure and to people adjudged by a physician to be obese through equipment maintaining constant levels of temperature and low humidity. Shocks from summer heat and humidity alternating with those from gelid, near-motionless air are stressful to persons in normal good health, much more so to those grown grossly overweight or inheriting a proclivity to cardiac and vascular problems.

In the long run, control of air temperature in the home to assure ease of heat loss, adjusted to mimic the progress of the natural seasons, might well be considered as a health investment. Misuse of the capacity to manipulate microclimates is simply too much of a good thing. Rather than the "set and forget" pattern too many practice too long, conscious attempts to regulate air temperatures and humidity readings in terms of the external environment will allow moderation of unwanted stress without abolishing health-sustaining stimulation. The enervation of a summer heat wave and the exhausting impact of a severe cold spell should both be tempered, while change itself should not be destroyed. June in January is not really to be preferred to January in June. Artificial climates are no better for healthy humans than ersatz foods, chemical stimulants, or contaminated air and water. Building your best body weather is not effected by destroying climate, but by ameliorating your environment.

Until biometeorologists and medical scientists are better informed concerning the sympathetic associations between change in atmospheric pressure, *per se*, and human tissue, organ, and systems responses, all we can do is make the air that touches our bodies warmer or cooler, more moist or dryer. It is unlikely, within this generation, that many persons anywhere will live, work, and re-create themselves inside spaces under constant atmospheric pressures adjudged to be most health-sustaining. It seems not unlikely that future decades will bring better information about the effects of climate and weather on human health, without necessarily providing individuals with the capacity to alter the atmospheric pressure of the new microclimates. For the foreseeable future, those who can and will are likely to migrate to health-sustaining regions, while those who cannot or will not may improve their body weather by informed utilization of standard equipment.

The single piece of equipment standard to all humans is the body they were born with. We seem to be learning, once again, the truth in the phrase "natural is best," but it is naive to expect any technologically oriented society to work toward a natural existence within a natural environment. The usefulness of inventions tends to maintain them, even when some unwanted side effects have been proved dangerous. Historically, humans have not sought progress through deliberate retrogression, or by abandoning convenience and comfort. Some of the contemporary nostalgia for the old-fashioned arises from anxieties of mind, not physical discomfort. The rapidity of change combined with the amount of change in recent decades has affected many with what Alvin Toffler termed "future shock." The human body has changed, too, but rather more slowly than the pace of technology. Man still lives, awake and asleep, with many natural rhythms: the circadian dance of darkness and light, the ebb and flood of tides, and the cadenced step of the seasons. The future, as much as the present and the past, will unfold within climates and weathers. Then as now, the most incredible of all machines will be the body man has been given and has grown. Although astonishing in both strengths and sensitivities, the human body will never dominate the environment upon which it so depends.

# 2

# Climates, Weather, and Mood

The record of human accomplishments is related to climate and therefore to weather to such a degree that until quite recently most people thought of a concept like "culture" as restricted to temperate zone peoples. The earliest dated examples of human artifacts and art works had been found by northerners in northern locations. Northerners wrote them up for other cool-climate readers and a neat sort of cycle sustained the awareness and pride of Western Europeans and their descendants in the continent of North America. Recent discoveries by archaeologists and anthropologists such as fossil skulls in Central Africa and massive stone structures in Nigeria, carbon-dated and known to be older than comparable fortress-temples located anywhere else, have encouraged us to rethink this view, without fundamentally changing accepted theories of climate as affecting human energy and accomplishment. As a species, man appears to have evolved over millions of years, not just tens of thousands. Man began to differentiate from apes in Africa, migrating north much later. The sophisticated artifacts, crafts, and architectural accomplishments of ancient man have been correlated with other evidence, all of which indicates that torrid desert areas today were markedly cooler and more lushly green tens of thousands of years ago. Then, the climate supported and sustained human activity. Now, the same areas discourage the commitment of energy to anything above the level of bare subsistence.

Humans dwelling for generations within temperate and stimulating climates have invented amazingly complex systems of manufacture, transportation, and communication. Permitted an excess of energy, cool-climate humans have also invented efficient and subtle ways of diffusing their own sense of purpose, substituting data-accumulation for wisdom, and exploiting each other's emotions. Since it suited their ends, temperate-zone men created, lost, and recreated an increasingly sophisticated technology directed to moderating the extreme discomforts of climate and reducing the hazard and inconvenience of weather that interfered with work or recreation.

Modern man can heat or cool the air around him, create or deflect sound, convert energy from one form to another and back again, displace mass, enclose or span space, and fabricate plausible illusions of what he likes to call "reality." He can add or remove water from air. Through chemicals, man can alter some interior life-processes and prolong a life threatened by disease. He has been much less successful in preventing the onset of illness or increasing human health for the individual or the mass. Humans have tended to concentrate on the standard or the typical and to achieve, whenever possible, the grand or the dramatic. The average, the mundane, or the modest does not attract and long hold the focused energy of the achievement-oriented human being.

A convenience- and comfort-seeking human is not necessarily a more civilized being. The capacity of temperate-zone man to damage and destroy has been nearly as great as his ability to create and control. Technological apparatus has extended the manipulative reach of the human hand, sometimes with unhappy results. Wealth has proved to be no special blessing, and power has failed to inspire grace. By increasing the range and impacts of the new artificial microclimates that enclose him, temperate-zone man has made himself the willing prisoner and seldom-complaining victim of his own energy, initiative, and skills. A comfort-seeker may be only dimly aware of beauty, dumb in the face of the unpredicted, and deaf to the sorrows of his fellows. A vital, energetic human determined to increase the convenience of his own existence can, by generating feedback that serves to nourish his pride, come to believe that since he owns much, he deserves all. Having confused motion with improvement and bulk with value, he often seems caught by the inertia of his own plunge through time. The self-praised master of what, which, how, and when, he is able to supply only slogans when the curious ask: why?

That energy-exchange systems developed and distributed by temperate-zone man have served to solve many local problems for short durations is without question. However, the more man learns about the physical universe external to him, the less, relatively speaking, he understands of internal facts. As our textbooks, research clinics, and data banks supply more statistically supported information—including facts about the human body, its systems, subsystems, disfunctions, and diseases—the more we appear to fulfill Ralph Waldo Emerson's definition of the expert: "One who knows more and more about less and less."

Perhaps we have evolved intellectually into creatures accustomed to externalizing information. Once pushed outside ourselves and labeled with language, any new fact can be analyzed, explicated, dissected into its smallest components, and disregarded. There seems to be a decreasing amount of art in our ideas, together with an augmentation of systems. Energy relentlessly consumed in computer-assisted achievement shows, historically, that it promises little in the way of natural health or normal joy. Progress does not make our dreams come true, but rather causes us to discard them as impractical.

## WEATHER AND AMBITION

You know from your own experience that your energy output, what you can do and what you will do, varies from day to day. A prime contributing factor to human ambition, and the moods that support or depress it, is weather. Granting that it is difficult in contemporary society to separate learned responses to cultural conditioning from spontaneous responses to natural forces, it remains self-evident that hot, humid days make the body's necessary heat loss more difficult than during periods of cool, dry weather. Most of the work that we can do or even plan is limited to cooling our metabolic machinery. We maintain, rather than make. Under optimum conditions which require less expenditure of energy for cooling, the surplus is ours to utilize as we will. Typically, our bodies tend to be self-regulating, with several sympathetic systems which operate in times of emergency.

## STRESS

Artificial manipulation of temperature, humidity, and the circadian rhythm of life unnaturally increases and prolongs what medical science terms *stress*. This should be considered a physical concept, rather than accepted as a propaganda device to spur sales of analgesic compounds such as aspirin, or so-called tranquilizers. In the physical, scientific sense, stress is measurable force or a combination of forces applied to a body at rest or in motion or a portion thereof. Muscle tissue is stressed by extension and flexing. The elastic capacity of muscle is finite; it can be stressed to the point where the tissue loses its capacity to contract. The force of gravity is a major, constant stress upon the whole body, but a fairly wide range of other forces are natural to the human condition. Torsion, frictions and checks, relative heat or cold, and increase or decrease of internal or external pressures all affect energy reserve and output, gross physical achievement, and rate of accomplishment and trigger sympathetic responses lodged in instincts and memory. These responses give rise, in turn, to anticipations and emotions such as pride, joy, anger, frustration, and despair.

"Stress," when used in drug advertisements, really is no more than a debased form of distress or periodic anxiety. Most advertising devices are deceptive in that they promise much for little. Drug compounds that relieve true stress are few; certain relaxants affect muscle tissues, diuretics reduce hydraulic pressure against the walls of cells, and highly specialized compounds reduce the force exerted against vascular walls and heart-valve tissues.

Stimulation activates the forces that stress the human body, and insofar as exercise promotes muscle tone, respiration, digestion, and normal organ functions, this is very good and no worse, usually, than mildly fatiguing. After exercise from work or active play, we feel "tired" but "good." Severe stress, on the other hand, limits or terminates ambition and can provoke tearful emotional collapse or clinical states of shock.

Generally speaking, humans have the capacity to endure stress for brief intervals spaced between rehabilitating rest. Response to stress is instinctive, automatic, and remarkably efficient. A perceived danger triggers an adrenal flow releasing abnormal, sometimes superhuman amounts of energy to muscle tissues. Previously unknown strength, capacity, and agility are exhibited in feats that surprise even their performers. Emotions, too, peak at extraordinary levels of intensity or seem exquisitely prolonged. Not all these emotions are primitive or bestial. Stimulation in response to severe stress provokes exalted responses and spiritual transfigurations.

Each brief interval of severe stress is followed by a "let-down" as the complex of musculature, hormone secretions, and metabolic overdrive returns to normal standards. The next set of stressful impacts is likely to produce diminished responses and measurably less efficiency. Still, a human specially trained exhibits an awesome capacity to endure stress that could disable or cripple him, permitted only moments or seconds during which oxygen intake and cardiac capacity combine to replace depleted energy resources and emotional balance. Professional athletes and people racing against time display this capacity. A source of vicarious pleasure to man has long been observing other humans in voluntary (or involuntary) participation in rituals, ranging from the mildly stimulating to the breaking points of flesh and spirit.

Prolonged severe stress is extremely damaging to the human body. Stress measurable as "moderate" which must be endured for lengthy intervals causes system breakdown, organ disfunction and damage, tissue debilitation or destruction, and disorientation of the senses with accompanying emotional trauma. The modern world tends to force prolonged periods of moderate stress on the average, untrained man or woman as a condition of existence. This situation is worsened by those manipulations seeking to create and sustain climatic or weather conditions favorable to accomplishment at the expense of physical and mental well-being. Moreover, as modern technology continues its relentless advance, the number of stressful microclimates proliferates, the facility with which moderate or even mild stress can be prolonged increases, and the humans affected are pushed closer to physical and emotional exhaustion. It has been suggested, many times in many tongues, that sophisticated diagnostic methods and measurement instruments alone are not responsible for record-breaking levels of infectious and degenerative diseases. Rather the actual incidence of cardiovascular disorders, cancer, gross metabolic disfunctions, avoidable accidents, and mental illness is increasing out of proportion to population growth. More North Americans fall prey to certain diseases, in some cases at younger ages, remain beyond the reach of known therapies, and die prematurely than was the case a decade, a generation, a century ago. In qualification, it should be stated that human health on the continent, overall, has improved slightly, due to increased efficiency of antibiotics in controlling infectious disease and mandatory inoculation or oral immunization against the child-killers: diphtheria, rubella, polio, and less well-publicized illnesses.

Mild or moderate stress engineered from stoked and forced-draught levels of combustion sustained hour after hour will cause physical and mental breakdown. The amount of energy artificially stimulated is seldom used in physical activity. High levels of energy, the result of adequate diet and weather changes within a temperate zone, have tended to become transformed into human exuberance. Practically speaking, excess human energy is "wasted," expended on activities devoid of profit or gain. It is flung off by men and women to make the pleasing noises they call music, to celebrate the body and the mind in dance, drama, and religious festivals. Since natural climatic habitat serves, internationally, as the elemental and therefore dominant factor of human existence, then *where* we live, must determine to a large degree *how* we live, which helps to delineate in time how *long* we shall or might live. Once healthful degrees of stimulation through change are replaced by standard and often involuntary intervals which call up physical and emotional responses, too seldom released in exuberant self-pleasing, we must predictably endure patterns of bad body weather.

## HUMIDITY AND MOOD

It is true beyond quibble that the old saying "It's not the heat, it's the humidity" summarizes the natural relationship between the dampness in the air and human mood. The amount of water suspended in the air slows the process of heat radiation and delays the rate of sweat evaporation. Little energy surplus is left for work. Even sprawled in a hammock, our hearts must work hard, pushing the blood to the surface of the skin. Humid, still weather is not only physically discomforting but is, for most humans, an unpleasant mental or emotional experience, aggravated when prolonged. Because the water-saturated air cannot accept sweat accumulated on the skin surface, annoying dampness creates internal sensations of suffocation or at least oppression.

Since humidity is measured as the percentage of moisture in the air in relation to the total amount of moisture the air could hold at the same temperature, a reading of 100 percent humidity indicates complete saturation. On such days, we endure moisture double that we can comfortably experience. Humidity of between 40 and 50 percent is ideal, and most humans "feel good" living within air holding no more than half its potential cargo of vaporized water (Diehl, 189).

The depressed mood caused by high humidity actually serves as a safeguard against heat exhaustion, cramps, and sunstroke. High temperatures, combined with moderate humidity, on the other hand, can be very dangerous. Suppose the temperature is in the 90-degree range, but the humidity is a comfortable fifty percent. A great day for baseball, tennis, or the beach, we think. We ignore the warning signs from our emergency system, profuse sweating, because our perspiration evaporates easily. Then, a mood-swing issues another warning: an attack of the "blahs," a plunge into the sensation of fatigue that seems to have little relationship to the amount of work or play already accomplished, perhaps in no more than an hour. Body responses include dizziness, headache, and nausea. Muscle cramps in the abdomen, lower legs, and forearms can result from sudden loss of sodium and other chemicals through profuse sweating. A severely stressed human—especially if elderly, obese, or suffering from heart disease—can collapse, unconscious, with an extremely rapid pulse rate but curiously dry skin. This is sunstroke and requires immediate medical care, usually in a hospital. The moisture-induced mood of lassitude is one we should heed.

The long stretches of high humidity in a subtropical summer season condition our systems to compensate in healthful ways. Unconsciously as well as consciously, we avoid stress and physical exertion. Relatively simple chores take longer to complete. Heavy rich foods no longer seem so palatable. We slow the pace at which we live, actually increasing our relative efficiency as machines. We convert to moderate slow burning of reduced amounts of food-fuels during active hours. It is like driving a car at thirty miles per hour for ten hours on ten gallons of gasoline, rather than speeding at sixty for five hours, burning fifteen gallons of fuel. We can get where we want to go, and more cheaply, too. But it takes more time.

The home air conditioning unit reduces the moisture content of air on hot humid days. If the equipment is set ten degrees lower than external temperature and humidity is not permitted to fall below fifty percent, it is likely that our work-day productivity will remain close to our best standard. There is no wisdom in exceeding healthful levels of manipulation, any more than there is in ignoring the moods that humidity induces. If too much change is made to last too long, the results can be damaging both physically and mentally. New moods of resentment arise in us; we feel exploited rather than "pooped," and are likely to transfer the blame for our sensation of being pushed to the nearest human, a coworker or family member. In work situations, we hesitate to exhibit some of our moods. We bottle up the feeling of being pushed, for fear that a supervisor will consider us lazy, or that worst of crimes, "hard to get along with."

This learned response to a mood is also unhealthy, for there is evidence that emotions repressed or strangled for long periods are associated with a variety of heart diseases.

## HOW HUMAN BODY RHYTHMS CHANGE
## WITH THE SEASONS

Do people who "blow up" live better or longer? A simple answer is difficult, but some evidence does exist that suggests high degrees of self-control exact a penalty. Many "calm, cool, and collected" persons suffer from hypertension and may be training themselves for future problems. Like the "set and forget" school of artificial climate users, they have a single adjustment and by failing to give vent or expression to moods of frustration they are behaving in a dangerously unnatural manner. It is not good to fight or oppose moods induced by artificial constraints or stimulations. Good body weather is self-aware adjustment to change, not the deliberate destruction of the seasons of the year or teeth-clenched suppression of moods caused or sustained by environmental conditions.

Seasonal change in the level of normal blood pressure for native-born inhabitants of cool climates is common and regular. Alteration in blood pressure can be dramatic, as much as a 30 percent measured difference between the highest levels during the winter and the lows of the summer season (Mills, 18). Given the nature of the new microclimates which concentrate massive artificial conditioning factors on urban man, it is difficult to get "pure" evidence on human health conditions. The use of hospital patients, prisoners, and volunteers has revealed that human body temperature, chemical composition, pulse speed, and volume of circulating blood all have a measurable circadian rhythm. It has been established that longer cycles of biological rhythms exist, too, some roughly corresponding to lunar cycles or moon phases, while others appear to extend for periods approximating three months. The popularization of medical information invariably leads to oversimplifications. Charting of "biorhythms" as now practiced, while based on laboratory and research data, employs crude categories such as "physical," "emotional," and "intellectual" that resist definition. The individual assesses what he takes to be his emotional peaks and lows. That is, the student-practitioner of "biorhythm" decides what such vague generalities as "governing sensibility," "nerves," and "cheerfulness" mean (unaided by internationally accepted definitions) and grades himself (without a standard index or objective check) along the

Blue sine-curve of his Cyclgraf (U.S. Patent Pending), marketed by Biorhythm Computers, Inc. To any doctor and to many interested readers, there seems to be, in all of this, much less than meets the eye. A pseudoscience, at once entertaining and harmless, like old-fashioned phrenology, is frequently profitable—for the promoter, at least.

## Spring

The most-celebrated of human "ups" is the peak vitality tide during spring. The total environment nature wraps around us then tickles many pleasurable physical responses and mental moods. The longed-for warmth of sunlight after winter's cold, the delightful flow of scented air over the skin, and the sight of new growth combine to produce or encourage fresh expenditures of energy and powerful feelings of joy. During the spring season, most humans record annual highs of blood pressure readings, too, even in northern latitudes where the new warmth has not yet melted all the snow from the ground.

## Summer

The summer season, in its turn, is "good for us," not because it offers opportunities for outdoor recreation or because we associate it with vacation, but because it creates health-associated conditions. For persons afflicted with hyptertension, at least twenty million Americans or 10 percent of the total population, controlled utilization of summer weather should provide a period of rest welcomed by overburdened heart muscles. All cool-climate humans have been severely and repeatedly stressed during the winter stormy months of abrupt and sharp change (even without a fall of rain, sleet, or snow). The high tide of vitality during the spring follows these winter stresses. When the summer heat and humidity follow, human bodies need weeks of do-little relaxation in order to recover. Sustaining the energy output of April into August, when only "mad dogs and Englishmen go out in the midday sun," is contrary to our inclinations. Modern man, who has contrived to feel guilty about "wasting" time, concerned that others may feel he is lazy, throws away his annual opportunity for needed rest. He will not permit his internal body weather to correspond to the environment that surrounds him.

We continue to expand climate control, manufacturing a sort of uniseason to the degree we are capable. We drive in air-conditioned cars to bowl in air-conditioned alleys or to swat a tennis ball in an enclosed and heat-insulated indoor club. We eat and drink in air-conditioned restaurants and bars and sleep in rooms chilled as much as thirty degrees below the exterior air temperature with humidity dropped to 30 percent, too dry for comfort or good health. Instead of a summer season that would serve its purpose to soothe our minds and ease our bodies, we attempt to obliterate this annual quarter. We prefer to change change rather than lend ourselves to it. Our culture relentlessly urges us to do, move, consume, and spend, and the microclimate of urban existence facilitates this abnormal restlessness. Nature fails to satisfy us. We must sprinkle salt on the beer of life. After all, if it doesn't have a "head" on it, it can't be any good. Our ancestors spoke of "Nature to advantage dressed," that is, the environment modified or arranged to make it more appealingly pleasurable. This is quite different from our modern attempt to master or control nature. The modern idiom of life disdains the natural and will not easily submit to seasonal rhythms or accept the fact that the moisture in the air around us and its associated moods serve to sustain life.

Repeatedly, we demonstrate to each other that we want what we have learned to think we need. Convenience and comfort are not considered luxuries, but human rights. We do not experience, but "demand satisfaction." We refuse to relax, but insist on having "a good time." Nothing for us exists that cannot and therefore should not be "improved." By rejecting the controls and cautions engineered into our bodies and minds in rightful association with the natural environment, we have damaged our bodies and cankered our psyches. For us, there is less doing and more watching. Our activities are fashionable, trendy, and discardable throwaways: jogging, platform tennis, skimobile racing, motorized camping, and mass-spectator media-events. In the restless quest for "satisfaction" we can buy or install, our national mood in the summer season seems to vary between brooding boredom and unleashed violence, apparently in sympathy with moon phases.

The studies of Dr. Franz Halberg sought to correlate external phenomena with human moods. His laboratory mice registered annual rhythms, despite the fact that light and heat in their surroundings were maintained at unvarying levels. Based on statistics from the Department of Health in Minnesota, which lies within the V-shaped trough of abrupt weather changes, he concluded that deaths from hardening of the arteries peaked around January, while suicide attempts crested in May, the onset of summer in temperate zones.

## Winter

The cold, unsettled, stormy discomfort and inconvenience of winter days combine to stress the heart and vascular system in a number of unpleasant ways. Some of these physical states of being may translate into mental conditions of depression or hysteria, as well. Much of this physiological and psychological discontent accumulates, almost unnoticed, until the human collapses "without warning."

First and most obviously, the human heart must labor to maintain body heat against natural chill. We tend to "help" ourselves by increasing the amount of animal protein we consume, along with rich, fat-drenched pastries and the sugar-saturated foods that have become traditional with midwinter holidays among Christians and Jews and shared, rather absentmindedly, by persons of no special religious faith. Combustion rises, and we attempt to radiate excess body-heat into work and living areas typically both too warm and too dry. Very few North Americans actually work out of doors in the winter months, but we have learned to eat like lumberjacks. Since the increased calories are not exhausted in manual labor, we tend to store excess fat in body cells. A gain in weight during the winter is quite common. Every added pound makes the heart work harder. The muscles must move more bulk and the blood must be rammed through more miles of tiny capillaries to nourish fat-distended cells.

Incidence of heart failure, coronary occlusion, and myocardial infarction rises as the laboring heart beats blood through the vessels, sweeping loose bits of debris and mushy atheroma from ulcerated pits in the blood vessel walls. These fragments of clottable material are pushed along until they plug an artery leading to a major organ, the brain, or the heart itself.

Strokes, resulting from the plugging of vessels feeding blood to the brain, are more likely to occur when our blood pressures rise, induced by natural life-rhythms in association with cultural pressures or work pressures caused by racing the clock or the calendar.

The tough heart muscle slugs on, day after day. Blood pressures excited to high levels by work-anxieties often remain elevated hours after the employee has returned home. The heavy winter diet of fats, starches, and animal protein must be metabolized, often during the early evening. The incidence of respiratory illness rises very sharply during the winter, as we all know too well. This, too, burdens the human heart. We feel fatigued, irritable, short-tempered, even without the hectic pace imposed by ritual holidays. Then, human excess of all kinds is not merely condoned, but encouraged, promoted, and insisted upon. We cast off the few restraints we have, just at the season when the exterior environment is most strongly affecting our body weather.

A still-small group of medical scientists and practitioners do not completely accept the germ theory of disease. The existence of microscopic bacilli (while evidently involved in many serious ailments) does not, alone, cause disease. We already have our germs, so the expression to "catch" or "get" a cold or the flu is not accurate. The healthy human male or female plays host to tens of thousands of potentially infecting microorganisms at all times and never notices their swarming presence in the myriad moist little caverns of body tissues. Each day, we are exposed to hundreds of thousands more. If germs alone caused diseases, then we would all be ill most of the time. Actually, only a small fraction of the toal number of people exposed to infectious disease ever contract the illness. Most humans take no preventive measures whatever. The concepts of cause have become more sophisticated; the germ theory of regional, undifferentiated exposure seems inadequate. Other generalized causes must be associated. Dr. G. T. Stewart, professor of epidemiology and pathology at the University of North Carolina and a specialist in public health, points out that many viruses can be carried by the unwitting and unaware human host for months. Then, triggered somehow, potential illness becomes actual. Stewart notes: "The resulting disease is in fact determined by the host, rather than the bacillus." Disease might more accurately be declared as the result of a combination of phenomena and circumstances occurring both inside and outside the body of the host. This has an important logical corollary: disease might be prevented by correcting or modifying some of the variables both inside and outside the host. Antibiotics can destroy bacilli within the human system, thus effecting a cure, reducing stress, and promoting normal good health. By promoting normal good health and reducing stress, will we not be modifying or correcting the conditions which predisposed the human host to illness in the first place?

Much of modern medicine utilizes drug therapies for both physical and mental illness. The basis of cure is pharmacological, monitored with painstaking caution by federal agencies advised by boards of physicians educated at great cost to practice medicine as diagnosis and drug therapy. There is an enormous amount of money invested in the research and development of chemical compounds by ethical drug corporations, many of them multinational giants with annual earnings measured in the millions. Counterpoised to this tradition is that group of men and women who feel that medical practice should be preventive, who argue that information is itself a miracle-worker, and who believe that the human mind becomes vulnerable to its own moods (distressed) when it is "insufficiently fortified against assaults of a psychic nature" (Cheraskin and Ringsdorf, 24–25).

What regularly and relentlessly predisposes the human host to disease in all climates, under all weathers, within and without the modern microclimates? Germs? Bacilli live in various environments, too, but best within the host. Roughly speaking, the host and his germs share the same body weather. By correcting or modifying life conditions, human health can be promoted. What is no doubt the most widely read periodical seeking to distribute health-promoting information, much of it antichemical and concentrating on natural benefits derived from careful nutrition, is titled *Prevention*.

In the stormy, stressful season of winter, both physical and mental discontent can be reduced by preventive acts: moderation in diet and holiday merrymaking, adjusting central heating to around sixty-five degrees Fahrenheit, learning to avoid sudden chill by slow, deliberate acclimatization, and coming to understand the benefits of stimulation while preventing severe stress and its accompanying mood swings.

The winter season in temperate climates can be a prolonged horror show for staff physicians and assistants in hospitals and local and state police officers. As metabolic rate increases due to the stimulus of winter storm-changes, our body efficiency declines. The human heart and the other major muscles of the body function at the lowest effective rate during this period of extraordinary physical stresses and emotional peaking. Tonicity (the poison-rate from wastes, bacteria, and blood chemistry changes) is highest in midwinter, the time for socially licensed indulgence and gluttony.

### The Holidays and Human Health

In measurable terms, it requires more energy to bake cookies, decorate an apartment or house, entertain guests and be entertained, wrap gifts, digest feasts, and metabolize increased alcohol intake in December than it does in August. Environmental and cultural stimulation will enable you to do all this more rapidly in winter than summer, but you will burn more food-fuel in the accomplishing. Holiday preparations and celebrations added to climate stresses thrust our lowest health reserves into high energy-consuming activities at the lowest known rates of metabolic efficiency. It's not surprising, then, to observe families of all persuasions suffering as hosts to infectious bacilli, as well as human guests. Heart attacks and marital discord are by-products of meeting the winter excesses with lowered physical and emotional resistance. Children, too, are known to exhibit the symptoms of high proclivity to disease and distressing mood swings.

Should humans hibernate like bears? Perhaps such a timed withdrawal into deep sleep and inactivity is not possible, but a deliberate moderation can only do good. Should the major holidays be shifted to midsummer? Cardiac advisory boards and specialists in epidemics might well urge it, based on their findings over many decades. It would be too hot to eat too much roast turkey and pastry desserts. Cool drinks sipped leisurely would seem saner than gallons of eggnog, a particularly lethal blend of potent whiskey, refined sugar, eggs, and dietary fats. In high humidity, we'd lie around at ease, while any desire to frug, cha-cha, bump, and Charleston slipped quietly away. And our celebration of Christmas would be more historically accurate. According to Luke's gospel, the shepherds were watching their flocks by night, a common practice in Palestine during the *summer* months, when it is too hot to pasture animals during the day. The birth at Bethlehem most likely occurred, then, in midsummer, not in the dead of winter. The fixing of Christmas on December 25 came hundreds of years later.

Exposure to cold, against which mothers everywhere give repeated warning, may be a less important initiator of infections than exposure to people. Recent British studies, for instance, observe that alpine teams, who must endure subzero temperatures, diminished oxygen supply at very high altitudes above sea level, and wind-chill factors of frightening severity almost never catch cold, even when stressed close to the limit of endurance. However, three or four days of celebration back in heated living quarters with abundant food, adequate rest, and numerous visitors and well-wishers are likely to give mountain climbers the commonest of respiratory diseases. Careful training and preconditioning to the rigors of work under alpine conditions and deliberate, acclimatizing exposure help climbers avoid illness. The average city office worker, on the other hand, may be attempting to scale the slippery heights of corporation approval and promotion without concentrated training sessions. After the midwinter holidays pass, he is often a victim of physical malaise and emotional depression. How often have we heard or said ourselves, when the midwinter binge is done: "Boy, I'm glad it's over!" An honest emotion, truly heart-felt.

### Winter Stresses on the Human Heart

The net result of the interaction between low physical resources and efficiency and the overstimulation resulting from weather changes and seasonal social excesses is to raise the cost-per-unit-of-work done by your heart. Perhaps it is not, at once, "heart-felt," until the accumulated damage has been done and the bills for doctors, medications, and hospital care come due. It is quite possible that we may be programed from the instant of conception with a finite quantity of latent energy. Overstressing the body is like driving a meticulously engineered motor too fast. Inadequate preventive maintenance will permit the heart to wear out prematurely.

The work-load required of the heart muscle in a less stimulating climate is lower, provided humidity does not stabilize much above 50 percent. A behavioral psychologist would observe that neither external nor internal urgencies are so strongly felt in milder zones, and hence are not so vigorously acted upon or reacted to.

Cases of heart failure, when the chambers of the heart are so weakened that they are unable to pump enough blood to meet the needs of the body (as distinct from sclerotic-triggered heart attacks which cause the death of heart muscle cells), have been demonstrated to occur in inverse relationship to mean monthly temperatures. When temperatures are low, heart failure (and heart attack) is high. When air temperature rises in the summer, fewer persons suffer heart failure. Coronary fatalities from other causes also occur in the winter more frequently than they do in the summer.

As modern man has extended the period of winter-type stimulation effected by chilled, conditioned air in factories, schools, offices, and homes, the difference between the January peak and the July low has lessened, but the *total* number of coronary accidents has increased. The migration of hot-climate blacks to temperate zones has been very substantial, as has been the shift of Hispanic people from subtropical climates to the temperate urban areas of the Middle Atlantic states. Both groups evidence abnormal incidence of disease. Most striking is the appalling rate of reported high blood pressure within the black communities of temperate climates and its result: a death rate for black males between twenty-five and forty fifteen times that of white males in the same age bracket. Death from high blood pressure among black women of all ages is especially common, too (Ancowitz, 67). One contributing factor may be mood, conditioned by the sum of conditions within the urban microclimate.

## EMOTIONAL STRESS AND DISEASE

In 1974, Dr. Malcolm Carruthers published what he called "a light-hearted" account of one of the many theories under current investigation. The theory is that the combination of a high level of emotional stress together with a low level of physical activity deranges the chemistry of the body, especially that which affects human blood, and is the major cause of heart disease. In shorthand: Emotion causes heart attacks. Dr. Carruthers' "light-hearted" account has a chilling title: *The Western Way of Death.*

Most of us are familiar with the idea that disease and disfunction (abnormal states) cause humans to exhibit describable moods. In the pages of this chapter, we have considered that severe environmental stress during the extremes of hot, humid summer weather and cold, stormy winter weather also causes mood swings. Dr. Carruthers wishes us to consider the full range of emotional stresses, many typical of modern urban life conditions, as the critical factor predisposing the individual to coronary disease. He is not merely seeking to gather notice and acclaim by putting the cart before the horse: emotion before disease rather than in association with disease or following after. Although rather brief, his book is lucid and convincing. Since no attempt is made to include all factors and his announced intent is clear in the preface, his selection of evidence is no oversimplification as the concept of "biorhythms" has been made to seem. Carruthers concentrates on the artificial nature of the Western work ethic: the anxieties of achievement against relentless deadlines, the "domestic blisters" of home life, marriage, and family, the consumer creed, high-density urban and suburban traffic, violent weekend excercise, and the cigarette habit, all combining to produce abnormal peaks of emotion, health-damaging lack of physical work, and premature death from heart attack.

The Western way of life (and death) is standard to temperate climates and has been exported to subtropical climates along with the cooling equipment to foster it. As described by Dr. Carruthers and others such as Drs. Friedman and Rosenman, who popularized the concept of "Type A Behavior," it is most evident in the microclimate of the "heat-island." That is, the hurry-worry and "galloping consumption" of goods and services, the frantic pursuit of wealth and "a good time," does not exist, alone, as a single set of artificial conditions. Rather, our temperate-zone life-style is contained within and maintained by artificial climate and manipulated weather. The "heat-island" microclimate, itself, worsens the quality of existence, contributes to human physical and emotional breakdown, and seems to precipitate, by augmenting the depressant effects of humid heat, some forms of mental illness.

Carruthers' opinion is just that, a theory, and one of many. He asks for a hearing, rather than claiming that his view is the single truth. He, too, is well aware that simple facts, unskewed by a dozen others, are increasingly difficult to isolate for study. With many factors he must ignore, he sets the impact of climate to one side. Yet it is the one thing we can be sure of, even while granting that precise measurements are not easy to make. Winter cold and abrupt pressure changes cause increased stress, even if we are *not* actively employed, even upon student volunteers isolated in hospital beds. Severe stress from natural causes means higher risk to the entire circulatory system, independent of the dangers of infection through bacilli we host within our bodies. At no time of the year is the complex of anxieties bearing down upon the urban worker/dweller more obvious than during the forty days and forty nights from the eve of Thanksgiving to New Year's Day. At no season is the human metabolism at a lower ebb. At no comparable interval do we overload our emotional apparatus with such high-powered stimuli. Never at other times do so many North Americans eat and drink with such compulsive abandon. In this crest of many moods and severe stresses, more of us fall ill and more of us die than at any other time of the year.

But what about the urban heat-islands? What about the gradual warming cycle our planet seems to be going through? Is there not a scientifically confirmed global tendency toward rising temperatures? If heart failure and heart attack and incidence of respiratory infections decline in periods of warmth, then we must be experiencing such a slow decline. If warmth and humidity slow and soothe body and mind, then we should be able to observe another slow decline in mental illness. Percentages and totals should both have dropped in the past fifty years, for during this period we have records of gradually increasing heat. Instead of these expected down-slopes, however, what the records show is the decline of public health in North America.

## THE DECLINE OF HEALTH IN NORTH AMERICA

North Americans are the wealthiest, best-fed people who ever lived in the history of mankind. Yet a recent major document titled "Preliminary Findings of the First Health and Nutrition Examination Survey, U.S., 1971–72," published by the National Center for Health Statistics, appears to support random earlier statements that significant numbers of our people exhibit symptoms of malnutrition, even in families whose incomes are comfortably above the poverty level. Male life expectancy in the United States is eighteenth, well below that of such "poor" nations as Italy, Hungary, and Greece.

Surely a high level of emotional agitation, together with a low level of physical activity, cannot account for the fact that we rank fourteenth, below France and Japan, in infant mortality. Our medical scientists report abnormally high levels of full-term infants born weighing less than five and one-half pounds, up 143% since 1960. More people, many of them urban blacks, have been diagnosed as hypertension victims. The absolute number of such cases is up. Hypertension is striking both black and white males at younger ages, too.

The life expectancy of white American women ranks about eleventh in the world. An American woman twenty years old can expect to be outlived by her contemporaries in twenty-one other countries, including some nations we have termed "underdeveloped." Despite the very real benefits of improved therapies and sophisticated medical training since 1900, forty-year-old American males can expect to live only four years longer than a man aged forty in 1900.

We have twice as many surgeons per capita as Great Britain, and each one of them operates twice as often as his British counterpart. Yet the Britons rank tenth in male life expectancy; Americans rank eighteenth. Cardiovascular diseases, including strokes, account for over half of our national death toll each year. Include cancer and the total comes to over 70 percent. This at a time when health services employ 4,000,000 persons at an annual cost of about $70 billion.

A study group from the foundation directed by Ralph Nader called attention in 1970 to "deteriorated American health." About 11 percent of the total population suffer from some chronic condition that limits activity, happiness, and productivity.

As our climate follows the global warming tendency, physical illness indices, both comparative and absolute, should be marking a slow, steady decline. In fact, the opposite seems to be true. The social stresses we have manufactured to which we submit ourselves and our restless superstimulated life-style that is contained within excessively misused artificial climate controls have worked, collectively, to make a sorry and often shocking record. There are signs, unmistakable and full of threat, that some things have gone wrong, instead of right, as hoped for and spent for.

We have not yet undertaken the difficult task of carefully and correctly altering the life conditions which predispose the individual to illness. Afflicted by epidemic health plagues, we have regularly attempted to destroy the bacillus and then rehabilitate the victim, instead of focusing the resources of the continent to prevent damage to the host. We have done our best within a certain tradition of medicine which, while it has eliminated or dramatically reduced certain diseases, has not really worked very well for a great many of us.

But new theories are being made public. Increasingly we hear and see the words "abuse" and "prevention." It is the prevention of abuse that is the underlying thesis of this book on body weather.

## THE DISAPPEARANCE OF PHYSICAL LABOR

For tens of thousands of years man endured within an environment he could not manipulate. Modern man manipulates an environment he cannot endure. The unrecorded history of man is very long; the invention of language records very recent. From what can be known now of the remote past, it seems that much human activity was devoted to gathering food. That is, prehistoric man worked hard in order to eat, so that he could continue to work in order to eat, and so on. Considering the long span of millennia, the ability to store and preserve food surpluses is a comparatively recent human skill. The ease with which we can do it now helps us forget how difficult storage and distribution once were. Early writings like the Bible are filled with observations concerning natural phenomena of climate and weather and their consequences on human life. Flood, drought, and famine conditioned life and health, causing widespread and more or less continuous states of anxiety.

Modern man, living for the most part in or conveniently near the vast storage and distribution centers he calls cities, does much less physical work than his ancient ancestors. He eats more and more often, which makes his work less efficient as regards the ratio of consumption to output. The new artifices require man to exchange time for money, which he exchanges for transportation, shelter, clothing, and food. Except in nontechnological societies, the direct exchange of labor for food does not now exist. As the environment sustaining life has changed, the types of stress have altered as well. With the dwindling demand for physical labor, the nature of stress has become increasingly mental. Artificial life conditions have created life abuses with a new complex of anxieties that condition, in turn, our body weather.

Primitive man was equipped with a set of alarms, sense-to-chemistry systems which automatically and immediately prepared his body for active combat or flight. Human beings have not changed significantly in shape, structure, or biochemical makeup since the beginning of civilization. Instead of apprehending, comprehending, and responding to the threats and opportunities of a natural environment, modern man is alarmed by fears that his artificial environment will break down and imperil or destroy him. The urban microclimate seems astonishingly fragile. Power failures, such as the 1965 blackout which paralyzed the American Northeast, fuel shortages, or insufficient money (governmental, corporate, or personal) are the artificial disasters now added to fire, flood, earthquake, and epidemic. Modern man must sustain anxieties different from, but at least equal to and probably surpassing, those of his ancient ancestors.

With machines replacing muscles and protein, starches, and sugars more readily available, the total human accomplishment of a week in a North American city easily exceeds the material output of many nations, even of our own a century ago. Yet the hormones monitoring and maintaining our biochemical responses continue to function as before. We are prepared for vigorous, even violent effort against external forces that, often, have ceased to exist. The elimination of manual labor—hunting, plowing, planting, reaping, and storage—has provided increased leisure and new health-affecting conditions, too, abuses self-inflicted, but originating in the artificial, not the natural environment.

Two tons of intricate machinery propel an obese consumer to a vast, chilled hoard of foods mechanically prepared and often chemically colored, flavored, and preserved. For some pieces of paper not really worth the numbers printed on them, the shopper receives foodstuffs of dubious nutritional benefit. Declining value is exchanged for decreased worth. The cooking fire comes in on copper threads to heat a meal that needs only to be opened. Satiated, the shopper sleeps, while metabolic processes burn carbohydrates, making and storing fat to be released into the blood to conquer challenges that have vanished. Eating, in the microclimates of a modern technology, is not now associated with work, but with leisure. Eating is easy. It is work that is hard to find.

Human bodily functions are delicately balanced and have evolved in response to needs conditioned by the environment. If the environment is significantly or dramatically altered in a matter of a few centuries or less, a single blink of time, this precious and precarious poise can be disturbed with some serious consequences. Alter the climate and the weather will change. Humans, we know, have the ability to adapt rather quickly to new life conditions, but major adaptations forced on the body can cause diseases, once latent or of low incidence, to assume alarming, even epidemic proportions. Biologically speaking, man, like other animals, responds to irritation, externals that stimulate or stress the body. Like other mammals, he can exhibit mental responses, too, becoming the most irritable of animals. Stresses caused by artificial elements in man's environment may be a significant cause of human aggressiveness (Rosenberg, 169).

## HOW THE BODY PREPARES ITSELF
## FOR FLIGHT OR FIGHT

When emotion is aroused by the instantaneous relay of information from the senses to the midbrain, an automatic emergency control panel is triggered, exciting the organs of the body. This emergency communications network is the sympathetic nervous system. The results are obvious almost at once. The skin pales as the surface capillaries contract. A surface wound will now bleed less, while more blood is directed to the major muscles. Breathing increases and the heart begins to beat faster. Oxygen-rich blood pours through the arteries.

### Sugar and Fat as Body Fuels

Two emergency-response hormones are released from the adrenal glands: adrenaline and norepinephrine. These chemicals, entering the blood, cause the changes which prepare the body for flight or fight. Two fuels needed by the muscles are promptly mobilized. The first, more easily burned, is sugar. Sugar is stored in the human liver in tree-shaped molecules called glycogen. The liver stores these molecules, building them from units of glucose in periods of surplus. Adrenaline poured into the liver breaks up the glycogen molecules, remaking glucose which the bloodstream sweeps to the muscles. There, two things happen. Some glucose is burned immediately, combusting with oxygen to provide an instant surge of energy. The remaining glucose is converted back into glycogen and stored in muscle tissue for later use. There is a flash of power, plus the sustaining capacity we call stamina.

The second fuel is fat. Neutral fat is laid down in almost every part of the body. Its base is neutralized by three molecules of fatty acid. Norepinephrine splits up these reserve molecules of fat, separating the base and the acid components, and they are released into the bloodstream. Free fatty acids are a fuel for muscle-work, including the labor of the heart, now beating rapidly.

As a fuel, fat requires more oxygen than sugar to be burned. The abrupt flood of free fatty acids to the heart muscle, when too fast or too long sustained for that organ to make use of, can cause the heart to beat erratically, but with less effective force. Elevated levels of free fatty acid make tiny blood platelets tend to stick together more easily. Since these platelets are involved in primary clotting of human blood, the body is now prepared to endure serious wounds. If muscle-work does not consume all the free fatty acids, some are recombined back into neutral fat, while others produce cholesterol, the insulating material for the human nervous system.

The modern microclimate seldom creates the need for violent and sustained muscle-work. Elevated fats, over the time span of years, are deposited by processes not yet perfectly understood, but the long-range effect is to narrow the passageways of the blood through the vessels. The vascular walls thicken or "harden," and the condition can be identified as atherosclerosis. Stressful emotional excitement created by the environment, through the complex chemical changes made possible by the stress hormones, seems to predispose the individual to later heart attack. The ancient pattern of life was response to real attack from without. Modern life conditions make many humans vulnerable to attack from within. The contemporary imbalance between human mental and physical activity results in chemical responses no longer appropriate to external conditions. Unnecessary, unusable amounts of sugar and fats in the human blood promote the narrowing of arteries leading to the heart, plus the formation of debris and clotting agents that can plug the narrowed openings. Additionally, the level of blood sugar is seriously affected by emergency mobilization of glucose the microclimate human cannot burn off as muscle-work (Carruthers, 22–25).

## BLOOD SUGAR AND BODY WEATHER

The healthy human must maintain about one-sixtieth of an ounce of sugar per pint of blood. If there is too much sugar, fluid is drawn from tissues to dilute the sugar in the blood back to normal concentration. The cells from which the fluid was removed become dehydrated; the individual's sympathetic nervous system causes constant sensations of thirst, and often hunger as well. These symptoms warn a physician of diabetes, a disease which can impair the circulatory system.

The reverse condition, low blood sugar, causes the individual to react with mood-symptoms: extreme fatigue, depression, overstrong emotional reactions, and general irritability. In extreme cases, *hypoglycemia* can lead to coma and even death. Too little is as dangerous to human health as too much.

Sugars are mostly converted to glucose in the digestive tract and absorbed into the bloodstream. Insulin, produced in the pancreas gland, regulates the blood glucose level under normal, nonemergency situations. At all times, the retina of the human eye and the brain require a constant supply of glucose. We have seen above how emergency controls produce stored glucose for conversion to quick energy—which, paradoxically, the modern human is often unable to use in doing physical work.

Modern man has learned to abuse his own body's tolerance for sugar; by consuming too much sugar he overstimulates the production of insulin in the pancreas, which seems to work at emergency levels to lower blood sugar content to safe levels again. This *reactive hypoglycemia* appears to affect humans who overindulge in sugar-drenched foods: rich pastries, sugar-treated breakfast products, and large servings of ice cream.

Earlier in these pages, it has been pointed out that external phenomena are continuously changing, that weather constantly becomes its own next stage. This is true of body weather—strong or subtle responses to stimulations and stresses, constantly monitored to maintain those approximate states of metabolism, heat loss, fatty acids need, and blood sugar that we call "health." Mild stress is good for us to the extent that it stimulates us to operate at optimum levels of efficiency. As severe stress can be health-damaging, so can inadequate stress, a condition that has been examined frequently in recent decades, both in coordination with space-exploration programs and independently. Special understress facilities restrict human movement and deprive the senses of light, sound, and

72

gravity-pull. Volunteers report disorientation and exhibit increased sensitivity to pain. The understressed human may hear or see things that do not exist. The memory seems to become confused and even simple tasks become hard to perform. Insufficient stress is another abuse of the human apparatus. Lack of stimulation causes both physical and mental deterioration.

In the modern microclimate, some contradictory conditions exist, all artificial, which combine to damage human health. The natural round of the annual seasons is reduced almost to a uniseason; temperatures are set for those constants believed conducive to high worker productivity, but little or no physical exertion is required of most employees. The artificial environment is replete with new anxieties and worries, while the possibility of regular moderate exercise is nearly eliminated. Noise level in the work place is so high that sound-conditioned spaces overdampen the acoustics to the degree that employees suffer from sensory deprivation. Much work, study, and recreation take place under artificial illumination, while natural sunlight is denied. At a time when medical scientists are increasingly aware of the myriad subtle but significant differences between individuals, life conditions for millions are becoming increasingly standardized.

Biochemically we are not able to make the adjustments that the microclimates demand. The farther our artificial environment pulls and pushes us from the natural world, the more inappropriate our chemical responses become. Drug therapies can modify some unnecessary, unwanted responses, after the impacts have reached serious or chronic levels. Preventive medicine, at this time, does not effectively exist. The human is left alone to manage his own body weather, now understood to be unsynchronized with an artificial and stressful climate.

One of the effects felt by many living in cool-zone areas, either within or near a metropolitan heat-island which conditions them day and night, is fatigue. While a farmer, factory worker, or floor nurse in a hospital expects to be tired at the end of a day's work, such employees tend to adapt to the above-average stress affecting their bodies. Men and women in these categories, and others as well— retail sales persons, service station attendants, and postal employees —are more than usually subjected to the force of gravity, simply because they stand up for about six and one-half hours of an eight-hour work period. The office employee, by the nature of that kind of work, experiences an almost reverse ratio of activity: about six and one-half hours seated and the remainder erect or in motion for short distances. Yet one of the modern health clichés is "a hard day at the office."

The clerical worker's sensed fatigue is commonly caused by deadline pressures, job-related anxieties sustained for hours, days, or weeks with little surcease and metabolic activity increased to severe-stress levels. The harried office worker scrambling to process the ceaseless flow of paper across his desk can consume abnormal amounts of energy, while experiencing additional emotional tension resulting from collisions and conflicts with coworkers and superiors. Unlike the factory worker or floor nurse, there is no way an accountant or secretary can work into shape. Deprived of time and space which might permit his body to exercise into a condition matching work-demands that strain the coronary vascular system, dull the brain, and cause inappropriate chemical responses, the office worker typically makes regular use of substances, themselves unnatural, to help him survive the unnaturalness of his days. He may have a drink or two at lunch to relax or three or four cups of coffee daily to keep up his "energy."

Accountants were one of the first groups studied in seeking the health-relationship between stress and chemical overresponses affecting the blood. More than is the case in other occupations, the accountant's work is seasonal. In the annual quarter prior to the end of the tax year, the work hours typically double, from about thirty to over seventy hours per week. Blood samples taken in this quarter revealed consistent and often large rises in blood cholesterol and more rapid blood clotting. A large-scale study of American business accumulated more evidence revealing the damage to health resulting from competitive, clock-conscious activities combined with minimal physical exertion.

Swedish scientists have studied clerks and industrial workers, while a classic British research design examined hundreds of London bus drivers and conductors, over a five-year span. The drivers showed higher blood pressures and cholesterol levels and suffered nearly twice as many heart attacks as did the conductors. Differences were explained, at first, by asserting that the conductors got a good deal more exercise as they collected fares on London's double-decked buses. Actually, the amount of walking a conductor does is insignificant. More pertinent is the fact that the bus driver must respond hundreds of times daily to aggravation and fear caused by dense traffic, the common condition of the urban microclimate. Also, the British bus driver, like the Canadian cabby or the Chicago trucker, is likely to be a regular and high user of tea, coffee, and refined sugar, and will defend this habit by statements like "I need the energy" or "It keeps me going." As we have seen above, harmful dietary habits come to be accepted as necessary to compensate for environmental stress combined with underutilization of emergency-level changes in the chemistry of the human blood.

Reactive hypoglycemia with accompanying mood-swings to bitter intolerance and disgruntled irritability has been held, in the opinion of an official of the National Institutes of Health, to be affecting over 80 percent of the adult population. The stressful artificiality of modern existence may lie beneath the symptoms of more than one life-shortening disease. One prominent physician terms the increased incidence of human hostility "an acquired failing in the handling of excessive sugars in the diet" (Rosenberg, 169–70). Refined sugars are highly concentrated carbohydrates or "empty" calories, since when ingested they do not carry with them the B vitamins and Vitamin C required to metabolize them. White sugar, especially, demands that the body give up stored vitamins. This can produce so severe a strain that mental performance declines, even as the final blood sugar level drops below what the coffee-breaker exhibited in the first place! As long ago as 1937, Dr. Benjamin P. Dandler wrote in his book *How to Prevent Heart Attacks*, "The rapid rate of change in the downward direction results in a severe *environmental* change for the heart muscle."

Since we have earlier used the analogy of the automobile to explain the processes of combustion, energy conversion, and heat loss, it may be apt to consider sugar as the additive most people pour into their tanks in the belief that they are adding a tiger.

The continental addiction to ice cream and cola products as cooling methods during hot humid summer spells is not, of course, conducive to improved body weather. The actual cooling effect is more psychological than physical, and the "quick energy" or "wake up" experience of additive sugar is, at best, of extremely short duration, and is followed by reactive insulin responses. In seeking to ameliorate our discomfort, we inadvertently double-stress our bodies.

Humans convert almost 70 percent of all food into glucose, most of it to be burned like gasoline in an automobile engine and at slightly better miles-per-gallon than we get from the family car. But heat loss in a car is quite simple, while in humans it is complex. And, unlike an automobile, we function rather poorly on refined food-fuels. The ability of the body to oxidize glucose is reduced if the fuel is refined white sugar. Honey, the sweetener found in nature, is that which the human body processes most easily for the greatest benefit.

Dozens of diet and health books available on the news-store racks urge readers to switch to honey. Hundreds of medical scientists have offered proof that heavy consumption of refined sugar has such a negative impact on human health that the stuff should be considered a sweet poison. It is certain that this habit makes for unsettled body weather.

## FATIGUE AND FRUSTRATION

Stimulation and responses can be measured, but they do not appear as constant to members of a group and are likely to vary quite widely with any individual at different seasons of the year; that reflects to some degree climatic drive or depression. In shorter spans—a month, for instance—some variation can be noted. The degree of fatigue influences responses measured during the course of a day.

A lost tool that blocks completion of assigned work can produce anger in one employee, indifference in another, generalized, unfocused resentment in a third, but bring out a previously unknown "Rube Goldberg" inventiveness in a fourth. School teachers, who work with individuals and groups more or less at the same time, recognize the potentially wide range of responses students can make to any learning situation, but are often puzzled or disappointed to discover that nothing seems to "turn on" some of the members of a given group. No teacher enjoys working the last period of the school day, when fatigue on both sides of the desk has reached response-depressing levels.

Regardless of their school of therapy, psychiatrists tend to agree that bottled-up emotions, analogous to static electricity building up inside storm clouds, are bad for humans. A brief interval of stormy body weather is better for human health than accumulated forces, long pent up, which finally burst. When we are deceived, disappointed, or frustrated, it's safe and sane to "let it all hang out." Shouting and arm-waving is not really antisocial and is to be preferred in all societies above atrocious assault and battery six weeks later. The long-range effects of pent-up emotions appear to be most damaging to the person experiencing these moods. "Letting off steam," then, is an act of enlightened *self*-interest as well as beneficial to the group.

We may have an oversimplified image of frustration: the sour, set line of the mouth, the grim clench of the jaws, the reddened face and trembling hands, a general posture of combat. This rather dramatic set of behaviors is typical of human frustration responses to things: motors that refuse to start, pieces the wrong size or shape, or some external environmental force not subject to control. Frustration responses to people are often artfully concealed by apparent calm, a cool, detached manner, and suave verbalizing. Inside, the individual may be seething. Minority members especially are forced to learn to wear masks that conceal their inner frustrations and stormy emotions.

The course of human evolution has seen the lowering of opportunities for useful physical exertion. For thousands of years, agriculture mobilized human physical and emotional energies in the annual rhythms of planting, cultivation, and harvest. It was possible to anticipate disappointment, at least to some degree; too little rain would most likely produce an inferior harvest. In advanced technological states, few men and women work physically on a regular basis, earning their bread by the sweat of their brows. The mechanical and electronic extensions of human muscles, memories, and mental skills create a major paradox: millions are capable of expending huge resources of physical and mental energy stoked and stored within their bodies, but there is too little work for them to do. This paradox, the stress from inadequate stress, is a commonplace within and on the fringes of urban centers. Energies without constructive outlets are regularly cited by sociologists as a contributor to antisocial behavior among youth, what used to be called "juvenile delinquency." The lack of work, with its demands for articulated goals and priority-setting and its rewards in money and self-esteem, is burdensome to modern youth at all levels of society, not just the minority poor.

## WHY DIFFERENT DISEASES HAVE
## THE SAME SYMPTOMS

General adaptation syndrome was first described by a German physician who began his work, using laboratory animals, nearly fifty years ago. Three groups of white rats were selected. The first was warned, then given mild electric shocks after each warning. A second group was shocked irregularly, without prior warning. The control group was neither warned nor stressed. The first group, double-stressed, sickened and died before the second batch, while the control rats lived the longest. Dr. Hans Seyle wondered why it was that diverse diseases, so varied in the manner in which each attacked the body or mind, had so many common warning signs.

Why did not each disease trigger different, distinct symptoms? His early experiments confirmed his observations of human patients.

In later work with sex hormones, Dr. Seyle noticed a common reaction to hormonal injections: enlargement of the adrenal cortex and shrinkage of the growth-regulating thymus gland as well as the spleen and lymph nodes, followed by ulcer conditions. Additional tests showed that laboratory rats manifested the same reactions to a variety of substances and compounds, in fact, to injection of any injurious or toxic substance.

Seyle continued to change the environments of his white rats: extreme heat and cold, exposure to X-ray radiation, threatened physical harm. He systematically altered the fine balance of blood sugar levels by administering adrenalin or insulin. Always, the same reaction: enlarged adrenals, shrinkage of the thymolymphatic system, and bleeding ulcers—the generalized symptoms of the human body when attacked by a wide variety of diseases. The German physician then concluded that any stressful situation, artificially induced or created by environmental phenomena, would produce a pattern of symptoms—in medical parlance, a syndrome.

Further work enabled Seyle to describe the sequence of stages experienced by mammals exposed to anything that activated their emergency controls and sympathetic nervous systems. First was the alarm stage itself. Second, the laboratory animals tried, instinctively or consciously, to adapt to the life- or comfort-threatening condition or situation. Third, they reached a stage of exhaustion, exhibiting all the signs of extreme fatigue and systems breakdown, and became extraordinarily susceptible to disease and premature death. The body weather of the animals responded to a stressful environment. Unable to control their surroundings or to flee from the stress-area, they attempted to adapt. The adaptation enfeebled and exhausted them (Lewis, 51–53).

## HOW THE BODY MAKES US SICK
## BY TRYING TO STAY HEALTHY

It is not difficult to see the significance of Seyle's work to a consideration of human body weather. Like rats in a clinical laboratory, urban humans are born into, live in, and die out of stressful microclimates. Like the rodents, they seek to adapt to what they cannot escape. They show the same physical and mental responses, the same pattern of symptoms.

A fairly broad span of diseases seems to be encouraged by the human body's attempt to cope with threatful environmental stress.

(We are considering only those artificial forces engineered to manipulate climate and weather with the end of increasing human comfort, convenience, and productivity, not factors we could agree are social or cultural in origin and impact.) The irony is that we are sickened by our body's struggle to respond to emergency situations.

In this resistance stage, the hormone called ACTH stimulates secretions from the adrenal cortex. Excess flow of ACTH can disturb or damage cells, tissues, or other bodily functions close to or far removed from the area of stress in the body. Prolonged anxiety, repetitive physical activity such as piece-work labor against a clock, infection, injury, or sustained fear causes excess ACTH flow. The steady seep of adrenal cortex hormones tightens or constricts the blood vessels in the kidneys. In a single instance, this may cause no more distress than a sudden urge to urinate (the "fear leak" that Ernest Hemingway noticed among bullfighters). Prolonged, day by day, for years, this influx of hormones can damage kidneys or cause hypertension or high blood pressure.

Additionally, it seems that excessive production of the ACTH hormone, interacting with other hormones, can increase the chances of disease. An immunity that appears natural to a living creature can collapse if excess ACTH is introduced first, followed by exposure to the disease. Some medical researchers now regard chronic headache, sinusitis, insomnia, ulcers, hypertension, some allergies, and some forms of kidney and cardiovascular impairment as stress-induced diseases, as well as emotional upset or neurotic anxieties (Lewis, 54).

Hans Seyle's general adaptation syndrome has been generally accepted through confirming tests on laboratory animals. Medical specialists, however, are not always convinced that human beings are so much like white rats that all the obvious differences between the two forms of mammal life should be disregarded. Albert Einstein once remarked that "When you get a very simple answer to a very simple question, that is God talking." Some scientists doubt that simple questions concerning human health can even be asked; therefore, simple answers may be misleading. While no one yet has been able to prove that human immunity to organisms and conditions causing or closely associated with specific diseases diminishes or disappears under prolonged stress, investigation continues. The human body is known to adapt, within its limits, to both natural and artificial climate and weather. By unconscious and unwilled processes, the emergency controls and sympathetic nervous system respond powerfully though inappropriately to environmental threats. Prolonged stress is known to create excess flow of the ACTH hormone. Fatty acids and glucose are activated, as well, but not subsequently consumed by vigorous physical activity. Through this adaptive response to overstimulation, the individual is pushed to fatigue. Norepinephrine, the "drive" hormone, enables the body to sustain stress beyond fatigue to the point of total exhaustion.

When we add to all this the evident fact that we inhabit and work within increasingly artificial microclimates that arouse emotional responses without providing adequate opportunities for physical exertion and stimulate us with mechanically manipulated temperatures, we may thoughtfully pause to ask: is it not evident as well that we should alter our environment in the light of human health needs, actively making better body weather, instead of forfeiting the benefits of naturally-induced changes in our bodies to the economic pressure to adapt? Why, after all, do people live in cities? Because they are vast storehouses of opportunity and money. Why do people migrate from rural areas to the urban heat-islands? Because that's where the action is. Why does modern man shuttle relentlessly from suburban homes to the stressful megalopolis? Because the pay is better.

At any stage of human development, change seems inconceivable, even while immediate conditions appear to be past enduring. So long as the urge to earn exceeds the need to learn, man will submit, adapt, and suffer the consequences. When humans believe they are obtaining something as personal yet as vague as "satisfaction," then common sense and common purpose are tossed lightly aside. The thirteen-year-old girl eager to acquire what she understands to be adult sophistication will ignore the warning of the Surgeon General printed clearly on each pack of cigarettes. It is very difficult for human beings of any age to delay the urge for immediate gratification and to choose those activities, habits, and ways of thinking that promote good health. We are all accomplices in the mistreatment of our own bodies. It is unfair, then, to seek to blame others for our own spells of bad body weather. One who seeks to adapt rather than to grow, to earn rather than to learn, elects to endure bodily damage and probable premature death. We are pretty willing victims, after all.

## TEMPERANCE AND EXERCISE: GUIDEPOSTS TO GOOD HEALTH

Good body weather or at least better body weather can be obtained through careful adjustment of the mechanical manipulators of climate and weather—that is, by controlling the controls. This will moderate the external stresses on the body and mind. Deliberate acts of self-control are needed as well to reduce the internal responses that are known to be inappropriate to modern life-conditions.

One man wrote, urging his fellows

> at least after forty to embrace sobriety. This is no such difficult affair since we are all human beings and endowed with reason, consequently we are masters of our actions. This sobriety is reduced to two things, quality and quantity. The first, namely quality, consists in nothing but not eating food or drinking wines prejudicial to the stomach. The second, which is quantity, consists in not eating or drinking more than the stomach can easily digest, which quantity and quality every man should be a perfect judge of by the time he is forty, or fifty or sixty, and whoever observes these two rules may be said to live a regular and sober life. This is of so much virtue and efficacy that the humours [biochemistry] of such a man's body become most homogeneous, harmonious and perfect; and when thus improved are no longer liable to be corrupted and disturbed by any other disorders whatsoever, such as suffering excessive heat or cold, too much fatigue, want of natural rest, and the like, unless of the last degree of excess. Wherefore since the humours of persons, who observe these two rules relative to eating and drinking cannot possibly be corrupted and engender acute diseases, the sources of untimely death, every man is bound to comply with them; for whoever acts otherwise, living a disorderly instead of a regular life, is constantly exposed to disease and mortality.

The writer, an Italian, set down his thoughts between his eighty-third and ninety-first years of life. In the introduction to his collected works he noted of his own advice:

> It is a kind of regimen into which every man may put himself without interruption to business, expense of money or loss of time. If exercise throws off all superfluities, temperance prevents them; if exercise clears the vessels, temperance neither satiates nor overstrains them; if exercise raises proper ferments in the humours and promotes the circulation of the blood, temperance gives nature her full play and enables her to exert herself in all her force and vigour; if exercise dissipates a growing distemper, temperance starves it.

The Venetian gentleman, Lodovico Cornaro, was not overwhelmed with awe at the curative abilities of the medical profession:

Physic for the most part is nothing else but the substitute of exercise or temperance. Medicines are indeed absolutely necessary in acute distempers, that cannot wait the slow operations of these two great instruments of health; but, were man to live in an habitual course of exercise and temperance, there would be but little occasion for them. Accordingly we find that those parts of the world are most healthy, where they subsist by the chase, and that men live longest when their lives were employed in hunting and when they had little food besides what they caught. Blistering, cupping and bleeding are seldom of use, but to the idle and intemperate, as all those inward applications, which are so much in practice among us, are for the most part nothing else but expedients to make luxury consistent with health.

The language is rather old-fashioned, but the advice is sound and useful today, just as it was during Cornaro's time. He died in the year 1566, being then slightly over 100 years of age (Carruthers, 130–31).

These ideas do not appear to have great value if they are imposed by a physician, family member, or friend. Observation of environmental factors combined with insight is self-learning, the base of appropriate actions to foster improved body weather. Not all the injurious impacts of the complex factors making up any one person's life condition can be reduced or eliminated by temperance and exercise. However, since it is one of the marks of the artificial existence of modern man to submit himself to too much too soon and for too long, a determined effort to adjust diet and to increase physical exercise will not fail to create better body weather and to promote a long, enjoyable, and healthy life.

# 3

# Sunlight, Artificial Light, and Health

Until very recently, man was obliged to limit his activities to the hours of daylight in his immediate area at any given time of year. Human achievement was limited, in good measure, by the ability to see. Although the sun was worshiped as one of several gods—more rarely the only one—prescientific man did not surmise that the sun might affect him internally as well as externally. Early observations were made concerning plants, not animals. The sunflower and the "Jerusalem artichoke" (a weird corruption of the Italian *girasol*, or sun-turned) actually swiveled to face the source of light and heat. Other flowers opened their blossoms with such regularity that the eighteenth-century botanist Carl Linnaeus left among his papers a list of plants that bloomed, almost on the hour, between early morning and twilight. Pliny the Elder, the most curious of Romans, noted that not all plants can endure direct solar radiation and that some bloomed in winter or even at night. Prescientific man noted that the rhythm of light sensitivity for edible crops and ornamental flowers was approximately that of the natural day-night cycle. More recent studies

83

have established as fact that some varieties respond in multiples of twenty-four hours. Exactly how plants "count" is still being studied, although research workers are certain that light sensitivity permits plants to anticipate seasonal change, to initiate bud-growth and bloom, and to prepare for dormant periods.

Animals, especially birds and mammals, manifest cycles of light-sensitivity, although these responses are much more complex, since natural sunlight conditions animal life indirectly as it alters heat, air temperature, magnetic fields, and available supplies of food. Natural light seems to synchronize the physical activity of animals, especially the migration habits of many birds and sea mammals. Light-responsiveness also appears relevant to seasonal mating of mammals and the spawning periods of fish. Some animals, like many plants, appear to anticipate change in both circadian cycles and seasonal spans. That is, increased or decreased amounts of natural light may trigger hormone-flow, especially from the adrenal gland, before activity, rather than as a delayed response to light stimulation. Time-series studies of human blood plasma indicates that hormone secretions rise and fall in intervals less than twenty minutes in length, and manipulation of scheduled darkness and light affecting laboratory volunteers reinforces modern awareness of the extreme sensitivity of the human endocrine system to light as well as to heat and environmental stress. Since blind persons manifest endocrine rhythms that are abnormal—decreased adrenal flow and altered basic activity of the hypothalamus and pituitary—but which can be returned to normal levels through sight-restoring operations, it is now thought that some metabolic disorders are conditioned by inadequate amounts of natural light. Without natural light, metabolic derangement. With natural light, restored metabolic functions at normal levels. Light may well have healthful impacts on hemoglobin formation, the activity of the thyroid gland, and the capacity of the human liver to rid the body of toxic substances (Luce, 122).

## SOLAR RADIATION AND AIR TEMPERATURE

Natural light is radiant energy released by the sun. A molecule absorbing light becomes "excited," and can transmit this energy as a resonance, a reradiation (as in fluorescence visible in ocean water or "neon lights"), or as heat. Solar radiation affects all of life on our planet in various ways by its color, intensity, and duration. Humans, now known to have a variety of health-conditioning responses to visible light from the sun, react promptly and dramatically to solar heat. What we call "the temperature" is a measurement of the amount of energy developed by a molecule agitated into motion. When molecules accept large amounts of energy in relation to their mass, they move more rapidly and collide with each other more often. An increase in temperature increases the rate of most chemical reactions, a fact we have been considering in these pages largely from the perspective of internal combustion, human achievement, and stress-responses of the metabolic complex. The sensitivity of living organisms is to light and heat, usually in simultaneous correspondence (more light creates more heat) and seems to follow approximate circadian rhythm (Watson, 16).

Cold-blooded animals are controlled in activity by fluctuations in air temperature, but with mammals, while heat may limit activity to a measurable degree, it is also true that activity determines body temperature. A sudden chill depresses reptile slithering, but tends to stimulate human achievement. High temperature, while it tends to slow the rate of human achievement, does not terminate activity completely, and actually increases the efficiency level at which man converts food-fuels to work-energy. Body temperatures of some mammals (mice, for instance) rise and fall even when the temperature of the air around them remains constant. Since man is active during the hours of natural light, his temperature within follows the pattern of his activity. Men and mice share this mammalian life-pattern.

Since the intensity and duration of natural sunlight conditions the temperature of the air (at least in rural areas, if not within the urban heat-island), it does serve plants as a clock or time-signal to some degree. Change in light and change in temperature may be more necessary to healthy existence than we have tended to believe. It is not possible to "force" tomato plants in a commercial or home greenhouse. Nurserymen know that the hot-house tomato grows best if the temperature varies and no special efforts are made to provide extra hours of light. The commercial greenhouse tomato grower seeks only to approximate the light and heat of infrared solar radiation of the summer season; indoor temperatures simulate the rise and fall of summer day and night. Curiously, for tomato plants, any change, either up or down in a twenty-four hour cycle is beneficial. Constant conditions are deadly. Unvaried heat shrivels the leaves, stunts growth, retards fruiting, and can cause the tomato plant to die before reproducing. These on-the-job observations have been confirmed by botanical research (Hillman, 89). While men may be like mice, tomato plants are not like either; yet these three varied life forms enjoy optimum health only under conditions of change, that is, under those conditions we call "natural."

Yet, it is self-evident that one of the conditions of modern existence is work and recreation under artificial illumination. As humans have learned to manipulate heat and cold to produce a standardized "uniseason" set at seventy degrees Fahrenheit, so they have extended the long hours of summer days through the year and approximated the day by artificial means, even when their portion of the world has rotated away from the sun. A commonplace in technologically organized states is "night-shift" labor. Most adults living on the North American continent are at least aware of, if they have not experienced, continuous operations of machines for increased productivity and profit. Hundreds of thousands of workers earn their living under artificial light, while millions sleep in darkness.

## TIME-LAPSE PHOTOBOTANY

About forty-five years ago, a botanist whose name is still obscure began to experiment with the exposure of motion-picture film one frame at a time under standard light conditions for periods of weeks, months, or longer. Each frame served as a visual record of plant growth, fixed on the film in a single instant of time. When the long strip of plastic was developed, processed, and then run back through a conventional projector, a plant seemed to burst from the earth, career upward at breakneck speed, and pop into blossom or fruit. Time-lapse photography was an especially intriguing illusion, with the whole life span of a tulip compressed into a few moments. We have seen other examples, perhaps, a building that appears to construct itself, with windows springing into place as the edifice rushes aloft. If the film is reversed, the plant rushes back down into the ground and the skyscraper unbuilds itself.

John Ott effectively invented time-lapse photobotany, designing and applying much of the equipment he needed. Two of his early efforts have been seen by millions: banana growth from first shoot to fruited maturity (a project requiring ten cameras and two years of patient work) and the more famous "dancing flowers," happily cavorting for two minutes (a sequence that required three years to capture and the Walt Disney studio to popularize on neighborhood movie screens and the home television set). The flowers were made to appear to dance in rhythm with the sound track. What really controlled the direction of their growth-movements was John Ott's cunning and tireless manipulation of artificial weather. The flowers "danced" because Ott had changed temperatures and the source of light for over 1,000 consecutive days.

The truly curious are never satisfied; for them, an answer found raises new questions. By combining his new film-making skills with a powerful microscope, John Ott was soon able to record *internal* responses to light and heat, within plant cells. Usually, on the cellular level, so little happens so slowly that short-span observation might lead an investigator to conclude that cell response was minimal. By single-frame exposure of motion-picture film, Ott was able to capture a single cell reproducing by mitosis. Again, he had reduced the activity of weeks into a few moments of film-time. During this session of microphotobotany, Ott made the discovery that lies at the center of his concepts concerning the effects of light on human body weather.

## HOW FULL-SPECTRUM SUNLIGHT AFFECTS PHOTOSYNTHESIS

Ott was photographing, through a microscope, the reactions and responses of individual cells to certain compounds injected into their environment. The botanist had placed filters over his microscope stage in order to control the color of the light being reflected onto the film. His purpose was to create greater visual contrasts, to make the cell responses more seeable. What he did, of course, was to alter the wavelengths of light reaching the cells under observation. Ott learned, accidentally, that the *quality* of light, as well as the amount, directly affects the life processes of plants. Photosynthesis took place at full capacity only when the cells were receiving the impact of full-spectrum sunlight. A change in either the quantity or the quality of natural light altered plant growth in predictable patterns.

Ott's thinking makes a quantum jump from plants to mammals, specifically man. Humans have been evolving for milions of years. During this immense span of years, man has been dependent upon light from the sun. The conversion of electrical energy to light is very recent. John Ott and his followers believe that full-spectrum sunlight is important to the growth and development of human beings and the proper functioning of systems and organs within animals.

## VISIBLE AND INVISIBLE LIGHT

The human eye sees less than 1 percent of the total electromagnetic spectrum. Not much is known about the light sources at either end of the visible spectrum, the ultraviolet and infrared, but some evidence now exists which indicates that both the long ultraviolet rays and the short-wave infrared exert a profound influence on the physical and mental well-being of plants, animals, and man, that these rays are, in fact, significant conditioners of body weather.

Natural light from the sun is a broad, continuous spectrum with a slight crest in the blue-green range. Sunlight cuts off abruptly in the ultraviolet because of the filtering effect of the earth's atmosphere. However, the longer waves of ultraviolet do penetrate the atmosphere at intensities comparable to visible light. So-called black light is included in the longer wave ultraviolet. Shorter wave ultraviolet can be very harmful to humans.

## ARTIFICIAL LIGHT

### Incandescent Light Bulbs

Artificial light caused by passing an electric current through a fine tungsten filament positioned within a vacuum tube of clear or frosted glass is called incandescent. This form of electric light could more accurately be termed "heat light." It contains almost no ultraviolet, is feeble in the blue end of the spectrum, and produces its maximum energy in the infrared wavelengths. That is, the peak of incandescent light is invisible, but can be felt as heat. Incandescent light bulbs left burning for more than a few minutes become too hot to be handled with comfort; they are considerably less efficient than fluorescent tubes, the other standard method of artificial illumination.

### Fluorescent Tubes

A fluorescent tube is filled with argon gas and mercury vapor. A cathode is inset at each end of the tube. These cathodes discharge electrons when the switch is turned to "on." A flow of current takes place through the mercury vapor, producing an electrical arc, an efficient producer of short-wave ultraviolet concentrated at a particular wavelength. This light, too, is invisible. What happens is that the short-wave ultraviolet causes the phosphor coating inside the long glass tube to fluoresce (emit electromagnetic radiation) in longer waves, as visible light. Different phosphors fluoresce at different wavelengths, perceived by the human eye as colors.

The type of glass used in incandescent bulbs is standard although it is sometimes tinted so that when visible light passes through the glass bulb it is seen as blue, red, green, or some other shade. The type of glass used in fluorescent tubes permits the visible light to pass, but filters out the short ultraviolet produced by the mercury arc. The glass serves this artificial light as the atmosphere serves natural light from the sun.

## Germicidal Light

Germicidal light is emitted through a different type of glass which is not coated with phosphors and does not filter out short ultraviolet. Short ultraviolet kills many forms of bacteria and is so powerful that it endangers human life (Ott, 24–25).

## HEALTH EFFECTS OF FULL-SPECTRUM SUNLIGHT

Full-spectrum sunlight appears to stimulate and to sustain the fountainlike surge-and-subside cycles of the human endocrine system, those highly sensitive glands that secrete hormones affecting human biochemistry. Human photoreceptor mechanisms are not yet fully understood. John Ott feels that it may be reasonable to assume that some human responses to light are influenced by its quality (that is, wavelength or "color") as well as its quantity (intensity and duration). To assume that the component lengths of visible white light have only the functions of creating pleasure for humans may be erroneous. Color may be incidental, while wavelength could be critical. Humans have been preoccupied with color as a contributor to communication of emotions or ideas. It seems equally within the realm of the possible to accept for further research the concept that unsensed wavelengths trigger photoreceptor mechanisms within tissues, organs, or cells, perhaps modified to some degree by the temperature of the surrounding air or atmospheric pressure shifts. Following this line of thought, perhaps consideration should be allowed for wavelength resonance of drugs and vitamins.

When a human being spends his active hours under either incandescent or fluorescent light, his existence is conditioned by the impact of visible light, rather than the full spectrum of natural sunlight. Does he suffer serious effects altering both his physical and mental health? Does good body weather depend on receiving full-spectrum sunlight in various and changing intensities and durations? Do we need the impacts of wavelengths of invisible light? How harmful is artificial light, or is such illumination a satisfactory substitute for solar radiation?

At what might be called the midpoint of his second career, John Ott began to urge that artificial light designs be changed so as to broaden the spectrum of illumination. This should not be confused with increasing intensity or augmenting what we call "glare." Rather, it involved the attempt to reproduce invisible light, similar to those wavelengths penetrating the earth's atmosphere from the sun. Two major manufacturers were not interested in the results of Ott's research. A third firm retained the photobotanist as a consultant and was able, before long, to market a fluorescent tube in standard sizes that very nearly duplicates natural daylight.

In his intriguing little books, *My Ivory Cellar* and *Health and Light*, Ott details some specific health results from full-spectrum fluorescent illumination. The well-authenticated examples are indeed remarkable: decreased worker absenteeism, lower accident rates, and increased worker productivity. Evidence is offered to substantiate claims that schoolchildren function better, achieve more, and quarrel less when their elementary school classrooms are illuminated by full-spectrum fluorescent lighting systems.

It is difficult for modern man to imagine a place of work, a means of transportation, or a private dwelling open at all seasons to unfiltered noise, wind, and light. The ancient Greeks melted silica compounds and worked glass and most certainly had the skills to roll the molten stuff into sheets. Given their technical know-how, why did they neglect to set glass panes in the windows of their public buildings and personal homes? Was glass-working so costly that it exceeded budget allotments for temples? Can sheet glass have been valued more than the ivory and gold employed by the Athenians in crafting a huge statue of their patron goddess of wisdom? Or was it simply that the bracing but benign climate suggested to the subjects of Pericles that they had no need to bother with even elementary modifications of local weather?

Certainly no man needs to be a Socrates to note that modern man lives behind transparent screens. About one-half of the continental population sees through prescriptive lenses ground to correct vision faults. We observe the passing landscape through the sheet glass inset in automobiles, buses, trains, and aircraft. We school our children and work ourselves in buildings where the windows cannot be opened, regardless of imbalances that may exist between internal temperatures, moisture contents, and light intensity. We seek to protect our eyes from glare by tinting the glass we impose between ourselves and full-spectrum sunlight. Most evenings, most families watch the configurations of cathode tubes transmitting images against another screen of glass. We have grown so accustomed to the house of glass we dwell within that we seem to fear investigators like John Ott. People who throw stones or seem about to do so are not welcome in the artificial microclimate.

In recent years, Ott's pioneer studies have been honored by citations and awards from horticultural, botanical, and scientific societies (including the Grand Honors given him by the National Eye Institute in 1967). Through publication and translation, some important guidelines for the improvement of artificial environments, light transmission, and human health have been established, if not yet broadly acted upon.

Greenhouses, small animal farm buildings, schools, offices, and homes are now being equipped with a new kind of glass. The conventional product screens out ultraviolet and permits only a reduced portion of the spectrum to pass through. UVT (ultraviolet-transmitting) glass permits the totality of natural sunlight to illuminate interior spaces. For the first time since the glassless past, all the natural and health-benefiting rays of the sun can reach humans, plants, and animals inside structures. All the sun can come indoors.

## Sunlight and Cancer

Additionally, there is evidence which indicates that humans who wear vision-correcting lenses can improve their health by wearing glasses ground from UVT material. John Ott has argued, often in vain, for regular research investigations, carried out under strict scientific control, in the field he calls "phototherapy," the controlled use of full-spectrum sunlight either alone or in combination with other treatment systems on a variety of human ailments. It has been at this point that his work has been disregarded or ridiculed. What? Sunlight good for humans? Ridiculous! Why, everyone knows it causes cancer. According to many modern medical researchers, "Today it is common knowledge that excessive exposure to sunlight, ultraviolet light . . . and other irritants may cause cancers of the skin." (Diehl, 232–33.)

Nevertheless, some doctors believe sunlight may have therapeutic value in the treatment of cancer. In the summer months of 1959, fifteen patients at Bellevue Medical Center in New York City, under the supervisory care of Dr. Jane C. Wright, head of cancer research there, were asked to spend as much time as they could in natural sunlight without dark glasses or prescriptive lens glasses ground from conventional material. These cancer patients agreed to avoid artificial light sources and to refrain from watching television. At the end of the summer, those assisting in the program were able to agree that fourteen of the fifteen patients showed no signs that their tumor-growths had worsened. Several showed "possible" improvement. The rather casual setup, the lack of a control group, and probable violation of restrictions puts this incident in the category of "anecdotal evidence." It might be considered to mark the beginning of phototherapy as an experience, not as a controlled experiment yielding evidence subject to later confirmation.

### Sunlight, Egg Production, and Tomato Crops

What makes chickens lay eggs? Light. Through careful testing, poultry experts have learned that light received through the eye stimulates the hen's pituitary gland. A stimulated chicken lays more eggs per pound of feed than does a sister who dwells in darkness. An operating poultry farm pays a whopping electric bill, because the houses are illuminated both day and night.

The pituitary gland is the most important part of the complex endocrine system, the "master balance wheel" not only for chickens but other animals, including humans. According to John Ott, the endocrine system can be affected or the actions of the glands modified by the amount of light and the quality of light received *through* the eye, which is not the same as light perceived by the eye. Fairly early in his career as a photobotanist, Ott was led to conclude that the basic principles of light-chemistry affecting plants applied, to an unknown degree, to all animal life, but in more sophisticated ways. The characteristics of light received through the human eye would, most likely, affect human bodily functions *indirectly*.

Chicken farmers fear the loss of electric current. A blackout will make egg production plummet. Tomato growers fear virus. Tomato virus is a winter season plague, the scourge of hothouses from coast to coast. The virus is strictly seasonal and appears after long periods of cloudy weather typical of low-pressure storm systems. No matter how sterile the facilities are, tomato virus will strike. Once it has begun, the simplest, cheapest system of control is to uproot and burn the infected plants. Yet, when John Ott moved a few virus-ridden tomato plants from a commercial hothouse paneled with conventional glass to his own, constructed of ultraviolet-transmitting plastic sheets, the sick plants recovered completely, set blossoms, and produced a healthy crop of normal fruits. Another bit of "anecdotal evidence" that pushed Ott to question the old concept

92

that virus was introduced to healthy cells from outside. Could this virus, at least, originate inside the living cells of the tomato plant? What did this suggest about the traditional theories of animal disease?

The energy of light enables the living plant organism to metabolize food-fuels through the process most schoolchildren memorize as "photosynthesis." Light is significant in the combustion mechanism. What if this rather complex operation were disrupted, rather like the carburetor of an automobile engine filling the cylinders with a too-rich mixture? When internal combustion in automobile engines is incomplete, the motor exhausts dark gases laden with unburned hydrocarbons. The fuel, only partially consumed, is wasted. Harmful deposits begin to foul the sparkplugs and valves. In like manner, might not unbalanced or incomplete combustion in plants produce harmful, even toxic residues? Might not this occur if the amount or the quality of sunlight was deficient? The toxic by-product would correspond to the description of plant virus. Since it was not a living substance, it could not reproduce, but could be thrown off like exhaust fumes or, brushed by horticultural workers, be transmitted from plant to plant. Once settled, it could alter the metabolism of the cells it touched, so that they produced, in turn, more of this toxic substance.

Could the lack of sunlight in proper quantity and quality so upset human metabolism that the combustion process produced toxic substances, either thrown off or accumulated within individual cells? Could this stuff be transmitted by osmosis from cell to cell or carried by the bloodstream? If inadequate or inappropriate light characteristics are a condition associated with breakdown, disfunction, or disease, would proper light adjustments of intensity, duration, and distribution of wavelengths tend to promote better human body weather?

## How Sunlight Helped John Ott

About the time that Ott began to consider the complex of the common environmental conditions—climate, weather, temperature, pressure, solar irradiation, and energy conversion—he suffered the most common accident known to the near-sighted. He broke his glasses.

At this time in his life, John Ott suffered from an equally common degenerative condition, arthritis. His hip was affected, restricting normal movement by about 30 percent. He took aspirin, and was advised by several physicians to consider wearing a hip brace. It seemed that an operation would be needed, replacing the defective part with a plastic hip joint. These were real problems to a man whose career and livelihood depended on his ability to lug heavy motion picture cameras and projectors in and out of greenhouses, studios, and lecture facilities. Two such professional trips took John Ott to Florida. There, he basked in the sun, wearing dark glasses, like the other tourists and natives. His arthritis seemed to worsen slightly.

Ott tinkered with his diet and tried a variety of remedies, including vitamin therapy. Hot baths relaxed his muscles, but did not benefit his affected hip. He received injections of new glandular extracts. For the first two days, the discomfort actually increased, but this was followed by four to five days of improvement before pain and stiffening began again. He now walked with the help of a cane. His elbow began to bother him. Walking even short distances became so difficult that he rode and coasted between his home and greenhouse-studio on a girl's bicycle, not much more comfortable, but faster.

When John Ott broke his prescription-lens glasses, he worked outside in the full natural light of the sun without dark glasses. Abruptly, his condition improved. First, his elbow no longer bothered him; then his hip condition eased so that he could walk without his cane and without discomfort. The Florida weather was unseasonably cool but, wearing an overcoat, Ott remained outdoors in the natural sunlight. As the weather warmed, Ott was careful to avoid excessive exposure to direct sunlight and sat reading or writing in the shade of palm trees. He began to think about America's prolonged love affair with dark glasses. Perhaps they were little more than a fashion toy, popularized by movie stars and associated more with glamour than reducing glare. Tinted glass filters out almost all the ultraviolet, thus reducing the amount of full-spectrum sunlight the body receives. The characteristics of the remaining light are altered by the color of the glass and its opacity. This double filtering restricts the wavelengths of natural sunlight. The nervous system can transmit only the information it receives. Only the peak of energy conditioned by the color and darkness of the lens could be received through the eye and transmitted as a stimulus to other body systems. Did anybody know that the selected wavelengths in the dark green range were appropriate for man? What about the new "fun-fashion" colors for nonprescriptive glasses with the ultraviolet-screening material tinted gray, yellow, or pink? How much consideration had been given to restricted energy transmission to the human glandular system?

The photobotanist's arthritis continued to improve. He wore no glasses of any sort and worked outdoors in the shade for at least six hours daily. After seven additional days, he was playing golf and strolling on the Florida beaches. He wrote: "To me the results were convincing enough: that light received through the eyes must stimulate the pituitary or some other gland such as the pineal gland about which not too much is known." (Ott, 49.)

Given the nature of his work, John Ott avoided artificial light sources as much as he could. Previously a periodic victim of colds and sore throat, he now noted that these discomforts and disabilities decreased markedly in both number and severity. After six months of his regimen, he went to his occulist for a regular checkup. His prescription needed such a drastic change that he was recalled for a second eye examination. There could be no doubt; Ott no longer required the strong prisms to counteract a weakness in the eye muscles. X-ray plates showed a definite strengthening of his hip joint. The condition that had restricted free movement by 30 percent was gone. The combination of health benefits that John Ott appeared to have gained were most surprising. By returning his body to the environmental stimuli natural to earlier generations of man—lots of fresh air, abundant exposure to *indirect, unfiltered* natural daylight, avoidance of artificial illumination, and regular, moderate exercise— John Ott appeared to himself, his colleagues, and his own doctors to have worked a remarkable recovery.

## *Skeptical Scientific Reception of Ott's Theories*

To medical scientists and research workers, one swallow does not make a springtime. Thousands of individual experiences are reported as "cures" to general practitioners and health specialists all over the world every day. Individual stories—even the experiences of groups who seem to share the same symptoms, follow the same regimen, and report similar results—tend to be regarded as "anecdotal evidence." Humans have a cranky obsession with medical procedures, fads, and fashions. The intensity of anxiety or fear serves as an emotional base for exaggerated hopes and claims. While we may remain skeptical in some areas and quote the old proverb, "Seeing is believing," when it comes to experiences that touch ourselves and those we love or care for deeply, we may unconsciously reverse the proverbial wording.

The history of medicine itself is replete with instances when doctors, humanly anxious to see improvement in their suffering patients, made premature announcements of miracle drugs and astounding cures. In such cases later investigations were unable to duplicate or even approximate the announced results. These days, outright quackery is not common. Stiff penalties exist in most nations to punish those who prey on the gullible, and heavy fines and prison terms await those who perpetrate health fraud schemes. But some health experiments are sloppily conducted. Frequently, a pioneer study embraces a small group and begins as random information gathering. The duration of the experiment may be too brief or the investigating physician too casual in his own enthusiasm to maintain careful checks and controls. A careful modern scientist tends to doubt the evidence of others, even other doctors, and most especially his own findings. Physicians, no less than other workers, prefer to create and sustain high-achievement records. Aware of this tendency within, the men and women who practice medicine or do research in special fields tend to be exceptionally cautious about announcing "cures."

The public as a whole and individuals tend to be less prudent. Secular-minded people may scoff at the pilgrims who pray at shrines like Lourdes, dismissing this sort of faith as rank superstition. The next week, the very same people may embark on a "no carbohydrate" diet, brushing aside the warnings of the American Medical Association that such a nutritional imbalance is dangerous. They may rush to purchase over-the-counter drug compounds and self-administer double or triple daily dosages. Modern man tends to put his faith, such as it is, in science. Away with the priests and holy relics. Bring in the medicine man and the head-shrinker.

No medical scientist is likely to deny what happened to John Ott. No doubt the photobotanist's physicians offer their warm congratulations. But this does not mean that any physician or researcher would or should accept Ott's generalized theories that natural sunlight can help to alleviate the discomfort and restricted movement of arthritis, banish the common cold, and improve defective vision. Ott did not and does not claim such universal and dramatic responses to phototherapy.

A medical scientist would require, at the very least, prolonged testing under controlled conditions with all possible contributing factors being constantly monitored. Take 1,000 persons diagnosed by specialists and known to be suffering from arthritic pain and hampered movement of the hip. All such persons should be near-sighted enough to require prescriptive lenses of conventional material worn throughout waking hours. Move this little army to Florida and keep them there for six months. Feed each volunteer the same amounts of the same foods. Expose them all to the same number of hours of indirect, diffused natural light and eliminate exposure to all artificial sources of illumination. Let none wear either corrective or dark glasses. All must play golf and stroll on the beaches. During this test period, a staff of trained assistants should measure blood serum, urine, oxygen consumption, air temperature and humidity, atmospheric pressure, and perhaps a dozen other variables.

While all this is going on, another 1,000 near-sighted arthritis victims should be recruited, moved to Florida, and established in a program identical in all respects except one. They should be required to wear their corrective lenses and/or dark glasses at all times. Such a medical migration would be very costly, requiring millions of research dollars. At the end of the six-month period, all the data from both groups could be stored in a computer and then retrieved, so that every aspect could be exposed to painstaking comparative scrutiny by a team of independent experts. What might be learned?

It is likely that some of the volunteer subjects would show quite remarkable improvement, others would exhibit moderate benefit, still others would be adjudged to reveal "slight" gain, while the remainder would manifest no apparent change and a small number some measurable deterioration. Only if the first group (those without glasses) showed marked and consistent improvement and the least-benefited subgroup was still better off than the most improved of the volunteers wearing glasses would it suggest to the independent evaluating team that full-spectrum sunlight might play a significant part in promoting better body weather. Even at that, no one would care to issue broad claims or to publish a monograph arguing a strict cause-and-effect relationship.

To the faithful, longing for proof, support for their hopes, or even an encouraging word, this prolonged and costly attempt to confirm, moderate, or deny Ott's general theory would be disappointing. Medical and health researchers, like politicians, seem unable or unwilling to make simple, clear, positive statements. The public forgets that doctors deal in tendencies, not truths. They process limited bits of information, snippets of data that limited resources of time, money, and personnel can provide. Even faced with evidence that seems overwhelming, most physicians would move very slowly to accept the concept that human body chemistry is significantly influenced by the characteristics of light energy received through the human eye. Perhaps most doctors would hesitate before accepting the view that light energy from diffused and unfiltered daylight plays an important role in the metabolic processes of the individual cells in human body tissues. All this might be "not unlikely." A more receptive physician might state that the elaborate test described "could be of some possible significance still to be clarified and confirmed to the degree that either is possible." An experience is not a fact to a medical scientist. The results of controlled and prolonged testing are not "truth," but rather information.

Moreover, medical scientists are not so open-minded as they would like the public to believe or as they tend to believe they are. Years of training—to doubt, to retest, to exercise every caution—condition the medical mind to *dis*believe. Certainly, this training and associated "mind-set" is a check or control for which man has every reason to be grateful. Certainly, too, physicians and research workers are very much aware of the esteem in which they are held by the general public of all nations. Medical practice has tended to be, overall, extremely conservative. Most doctors have deep, ingrained traditions of extraordinary prudence accompanied by a preference for the status quo and marked suspicion of the outsider. John Ott, who does not hold a medical degree, saw professional doubt and disinterest become personal discourtesy when he ventured to suggest other ways of thinking about cancer.

It is fair, although not always popular, to point out that as there are fashions in hair styles and apparel, forms of entertainment and recreation, diet and slang, there are fashionable, approved ways of thinking about problems and designing solutions. For example, if I am fully convinced by education and experience that a problem is extremely complex and will therefore require a complicated, rather slow, and probably expensive solution, I will not very readily open my mind to some stranger who says, "Why not just add a cup of warm water?" or offers some similar simple, quick, and cheap remedy. On the other hand, if my conviction is that the problem is simple, requiring only a cup of warm water to solve it, then I will tend to reject complicated, long-range, and expensive solutions, no matter who suggests that approach. I may be, in either case, right or wrong. To some degree, I will be biased, one way or the other. Education, experience, feedback reinforcement, personal ego, a sense of team membership, personal insecurity—all of these factors urge us, consciously and unconsciously, to reject new ideas. Even

*98*

when the new way of thinking replaces the old, I may prefer the past known to the now most-likely. Medical scientists are not immune to standard human patterns of thought and prejudgment.

The current and widespread way of thinking about the problem of cancer is that this major human health menace is caused by a virus or is associated with a virus. The solution must then be to locate and isolate the virus or the strain to which the harmful organism belongs. Next, find some substance that will kill the known organisms without damaging the otherwise healthy tissue. An ideal virus-killing compound should be safe and inexpensive to manufacture and easily administered by oral dosage, application as a salve or ointment, or hypodermic injection. Also, the cancer-stopping agent should not be too broadly contraindicated; that is, most people should be able to accept treatment without harmful side effects. All this is an extremely tall order.

Given the mystifying nature of the disease and the restrictions that must reasonably be set around the cure, the reader may better appreciate the practical and human problems that beset the medical scientist devoted to the investigation of what the public calls "cancer."

When John Ott explained the Bellevue Medical Center experience to the research staff of a leading hospital in Houston, Texas, hoping for a bigger, better controlled investigation of the impacts of light and associated body weather responses, the reaction he got from the doctors there was, in his words, "stone cold." In fact, he was advised to stop talking about what had happened to the fourteen cancer patients, since no control group had been established and maintained there, even during the few months of a single summer. Additionally, his procedures had not been tested first on laboratory animals, a standard research method. So Ott set about remedying the shortcomings in his research.

John Ott and Dr. Samuel Gabby combined their resources in Elgin, Illinois. Ott had the theory, and Gabby had 136 white rodents of the $C_3H$ strain, specially bred to be highly susceptible to spontaneous tumor development, that is, "cancer prone." The rats were separated into three groups, the classic division for experimental testing. Thirty pairs were kept exposed to white fluorescent tubes that approximated full-spectrum natural light. The second group of thirty pairs were kept in another room lit by pink fluorescent tubes of standard manufacture, the kind frequently installed in ladies' rooms, since pink light creates a pleasant illusion of cheerful good health. The control, eight pairs of rodents, were kept in a room without electrical-powered illumination. The control rats received only daylight, filtered through conventional window glass, the kind that blocks out ultraviolet.

The cancer-prone rats exposed to pink fluorescent light manifested symptoms of tumor-growth first. The second group to contract cancer were the rats exposed to the daylight white fluorescent light. The rodents remaining healthy the longest were the control animals, living exposed to filtered daylight. Significantly, the pink-light rats had litters of only two or three offspring, while the white-light and daylight groups produced from six to fifteen infants per litter, normal birth rates for such animals.

Ott and Dr. Gabby submitted a full report on the effect of various kinds of light on white rats to the editors of the *Illinois Medical Journal*. The report was not published. When an informal presentation was made to several members of the Illinois branch of the American Cancer Society, it stirred up a small local storm of criticism against Dr. Gabby.

The bane of any actor's life is type-casting. In publishing, it is "known" that poets can't write fiction and that novelists make mediocre poets. John Ott was type-cast in the 1960s. His time-lapse motion picture sequences had been incorporated into Walt Disney productions. Millions of persons (some of them doctors) had seen the enchanting and astonishing sequences in *Secrets of Life* and *Nature's Half-Acre*. A decade is rather a long time on the continent of North America, where technological advance is rather more rapid than elsewhere. By the 1970s time-lapse film techniques had become commonplace, both in medical science and the entertainment industry.

One of the problems of living within a culture that rapidly adopts, improves, and then replaces its own technology is that created by the accompanying tendency to specialize information and skills. Once you are identified and labeled, others out of convenience more often than malice adopt a mind-set, or "fix." Medical science tends to distrust the generalist. So do the academic world, business, and government. To be interested in many things and to seek to deploy skills in more than a single area runs counter to the cultural pressure to compartmentalize both ideas and people. In attempting to solve this problem, John Ott incorporated his nonprofit Time-Lapse Research Foundation and made application for grant monies to the National Institutes of Health in 1962. He was careful *not* to mention the Bellevue Medical Center experience. The letter of reply reads, in part (Ott, 64):

The application was not approved and the reasons given were: The reviewers believed that the proposal did not indicate familiarity of the applicant with existing research in the field, or with scientific methods in general. They recognized that you are experienced in time-lapse microphotography; that the films you listed in support of your request are of a very popular kind, but it did not seem likely that anything of scientific merit would emerge from such a program.

In so many words, the lack of abundant literature in the field was considered to count against Ott. Since he did not have an M.D. degree, doubt existed that he understood the methods of science. Finally, the tone of the letter suggests that to make "very popular" films was quite inappropriate behavior. Presumably, then, scientists should make extremely unpopular films, or none at all?

Martin Duberman, distinguished professor of history at Lehman College, City University of New York, writing in another context, recently observed (*New York Times Magazine*, 9 November 1975, pp. 69–70):

> Societies tend to produce "expert opinion" that clarifies and consolidates already acceptable assumptions about how the world works. Though specialists usually view themselves as pioneers driven by "the need to know," fearlessly exploring the frontiers of Truth, the typical role they play is to confirm, not challenge, dominant social attitudes. Only the greatest in each generation—often to their own surprise, sometimes contrary to their own expectations—re-examine experience in a sufficiently original way to unsettle familiar notions. And it's only with the passage of time that we're able to distinguish with any confidence between approaches that marked a genuine passage to the "newness" from those that—however novel the packaging—served essentially to rationalize existing arrangements.

Duberman's low-keyed summation seems a fair description of Ott's dilemma and of the problem any investigator must expect to face when the experts are members of the Establishment. For John Ott to suggest that eyes might be used by the body for purposes other than seeing and the most healthy light was unfiltered full-spectrum sunlight was a little too much, given our human habit of ringing in "experts" to confirm the already-known. When the photobotanist began to press industry, government agencies, and medical and scientific institutes for monies to expand the literature in an understudied field, he got nowhere. Corporations making window glass or artificial illumination systems had no public policies developed *re* ultraviolet wavelengths. Such manufacturers could see no special reasons why they should consider themselves in the business of affecting public health. In the early 1960s, there were no budget allocations anywhere specified to encourage study of the effects of natural and artificial light on plants, animals, or people. There was no great interest in the idea. There was, in truth, very little in "the literature"—published articles in accredited and approved journals, monographs, or books published by degreed authors of some renown—to spark any interest. Ott got very standardized replies, much to the effect that, Yes, we know that sunlight is natural and incandescent and fluorescent systems are not, just as we are aware that conventional glass screens out ultraviolet. Yes, we're in the business of making the systems you describe. Maybe there's something in what you say. No, we're not interested. No, you can't have any of our money.

Rather like conventional glass itself, the human mind is a kind of filter that permits the passage of certain ideas, but blocks others. Ott, his colleagues, and a handful of curious scientists were like ultraviolet, operating on a wavelength that was quite natural, but unwanted and, for all practical purposes, socially and economically invisible.

## MALILLUMINATION

Recent studies compiled by the statistical division of the Department of Health, Education and Welfare deal with the relationship between nutrition and health in the United States. Despite the fact that citizens of North America have the highest per capita income in the world, significant numbers exhibit the symptoms of malnutrition. In like fashion, publications from the United States Environmental Protection Agency inform readers of the health consequences of sulfur oxides in the air. Additional studies have helped to evaluate the potability of drinking water in both rural and urban areas. In view of these studies, and the nature of contemporary shelter, it seems reasonable to ask why no governmental agency or major scientific institute has undertaken an investigation into the effects of both natural and artificial light. If some Americans —black and white, young and old, poor and well-off—exhibit signs of malnutrition, might not a comparable number suffer from malillumination? Such a study might reveal that deleterious effects are more common among the urban middle class than in any other socioeconomic group.

Research so far has established as fact that the blind manifest reduced amplitude of adrenal and blood cell rhythms. Surgical intervention to remove cataracts from the surface of the eye restores adrenal activity to its normal range. The physiological importance of light to the nearly blind has been demonstrated, with water balance, electrolyte levels, fat, protein and carbohydrates, and adrenal hormones measured as determining states of malillumination. What is not well known is the range of impacts of inappropriate or inadequate light on normal-vision humans.

Very simply stated, the retina of the eye receives and transmits the light-energy touching it to the endocrine system. Light of extreme intensity is a form of stress; so is total absence of light. Precisely timed flickering light induces powerful feelings of annoyance and anger in normal patients and can trigger seizures in persons afflicted with epilepsy. If the amount of energy is altered by limiting the wavelengths of light reaching the retina, the endocrine system is also affected, although less dramatically. No studies have been made on humans subjected to this condition over long periods of time. The photoreceptor systems of man are judged to be sensitive and highly involved switching and control responses, all much more difficult to measure and appraise than with laboratory animals or chickens.

By pushing into this area of exploration, John Ott was able to make some significant contribution to "the literature" (lack of which had helped to deny him funds, as we have noted) and therefore to lines of investigation concerning human health. Interest and support came from a noted ophthalmologist, Dr. T. G. Dickinson, who pointed out that a layer of cells in the retina of the eye of an animal (known as the pigment epithelial cells) has no known function for seeing, as such. This cell layer is, however, highly sensitive to certain tranquilizing drugs. Ott's time-lapse photography techniques could provide a test useful as a permanent record of tranquilizer overdose conditions. This new idea enabled Ott to prove, through photography, that after continuous twelve-hour exposure to ordinary incandescent light, each day for one week, about 90 percent of these sensitive pigment granules became almost motionless, as if stunned into inactivity. When ultraviolet wavelengths in visible light were added, the pigment grains in the eye became normally active again.

What this appears to establish is the negative effect of the kind of light bulbs most humans use daily, year after year. What is suggested is that these sensitive cells are "tuned" to the full spectrum of natural sunlight. What could be stated as an opinion would be that natural light is normal and good, artificial abnormal and not so good, at least different, and possibly harmful over a long span of years.

How potentially damaging the effect of malillumination may prove to be on human blood chemistry remains mysterious. Does the absence of certain wavelengths cause chemical reactions or prevent them? If glandular activity is altered by artificial light, is the resulting activity excessive, deficient, both, or neither to a health-affecting degree?

A single example may serve to indicate the difficulty. Modern techniques of microbiology and photography permit investigators to make motion picture records of living tissues and cells. Instead of killing and then staining the tissues, the medical scientist often prefers to use a *phase-contrast* microscope. The bright light bounced off the mirror and reflected through the material under the microscope lens is controlled by filters to create sharp contrasts that can be seen easily. Green, blue, or red filters are placed over the light source. When the shutter of the motion picture camera clicks, exposing a single frame of film and recording less than an instant of time, some surprising effects of light can be observed. When exposed to red light, the heart cells of embryo chickens rupture. Is it possible that some wavelengths of solar irradiation affect unborn humans, too? Pregnancy in humans lasts about nine months, two full seasons. During this time, the mother may be responding herself to changes in light and indirectly affecting the life in her womb.

## EFFECT OF LIGHT ON THE MATING OF DUCKS

Most humans are aware in a casual, unexamined way that our eyes function for purposes other than seeing. The visible surface of the eye transmits emotions for which we have a number of expressive phrases: "a come-hither glance," "an icy stare," "a scornful, still regard," and others. Other, culturally conditioned words describe the eyes turned toward us: "warm," "cold," "steely," "calculating," and so on. Rage, suspicion, trust, joy, and sorrow are emotional states communicated by glances, along with gestures and posture. Body language transmits some states of emotional body weather.

A classic study by two French doctors, titled "The Control of Visible Radiations of the Gonadotropic Activity of the Duck Hypophysis," concerns the effect of red light on the mating activity of ducks. While the path light uses to stimulate the sex glands is not known, the retina of the eye is involved. Even when the birds are partially blinded, so that the stimulus of light does not reach the brain, sexual activity results from irradiations in the orange to red range. Even when the optic nerves of the ducks studied were damaged or destroyed, they were aroused by the effect of light, transmitted as energy to the hypothalamus gland. Other wavelengths had no such effect. The photoreceptor mechanism, at least in ducks, need not be in natural operation in order to excite both cell growth and some specific activities (Ott, 75–76).

Dr. Franz Von Hollwich suspects that light may play a role as a synchronizer of the hypothalamic-pituitary-adrenal mechanism that controls hormone rhythms conditioning basic activities, growth, and blood chemistry. Gay Gaer Luce, who authored *Biological Rhythms in Psychiatry and Medicine* for the United States Department of Health, Education and Welfare and The National Institute of Mental Health in 1970, offers the following opinion (Luce, 123):

> For rodents and for man, the alternation of light and darkness appears to trigger activity within the nervous system that in turn helps to regulate physiological cycles. Are there light sensitive structures in the brain that would respond to nervous information influencing the reproductive system? The pineal may be one organ that gives biochemical information to the brain and endocrine system about the alternation of light and darkness. Researchers on this gland suggest it may play a mediating role in a relationship between light and sexual function.

## QUALITY VIS-A-VIS QUANTITY OF LIGHT

All life on our planet depends, in some way, on the sun. The position of this flaming star, the disturbances of its rate of burning and variety of energy-release, and the length of its irradiated waves are conditions of the climates and weather that microorganisms, plants, animals, and man experience. All life, directly or indirectly, requires certain quantities and qualities of natural sunlight to grow, live, and reproduce. While John Ott and his followers are interested in the quality of light, the bulk of research work is dedicated to examining the effects of quantity. Fashionable thinking about light remains in the areas of intensity and duration, that is, the more "seeable" aspects of full-spectrum sunlight.

Man, like all other species, evolved through thousands of centuries, his stumbling and imperiled progress illuminated by natural sunlight. The invention of all present systems of artificial light is so new that very little is known of potential or actual health effects.

Human sensitivity, both physical and emotional, to sun flare activity is well documented. It is also apparent that the most observable characteristics of visible light alter the functioning of complicated glandular systems. Investigations, such as those initiated by John Ott into the effects of ultraviolet and other invisible forms of light, have raised some significant questions. Some change in the way of thinking about light may be overdue, since the present trend fails to take all factors of light into consideration. Future studies may well expand to include the quality of both natural and artificial illumination, not just their quantity.

It is possible, too, that scientists may discover some forms now considered to be viruses are really other substances created within plant and animal tissues by still-unknown responses that can be associated with malillumination. Orange to red light does seem to have the characteristic wavelengths capable of conversion and transmission to tissues and organs, specifically those glands most affecting human biochemistry. Conventional window glass and materials used for grinding prescriptive lenses filter out ultraviolet for millions every hour, every day over human lifetimes. Some anecdotal evidence exists which suggests that phototherapy has been permitted to lag far behind pharmacological therapeutics. Unlike drugs, which usually require symptoms of illness before they can be prescribed, natural sunlight, as a primary environmental factor, may turn out to be a major tool in preventive medicine.

The two most widely used systems of artificial illumination, incandescent bulbs and fluorescent tubes, do not provide for plants, animals, and humans the light characteristics typically associated with the healthful stimulation of receptors, transmitters, and mammal glands. In the words of endocrinologist Joseph Meites: "We have no idea how many diseases are linked with hormone problems, but we do know that several diseases such as diabetes, infertility, cancer and thyroid disorders are involved with hormone imbalance." (Ott, 78.)

The individual seeking to better his body weather may be well advised to avoid absence or overabundance of natural sunlight and to give some special consideration to the probable health benefits to be gained from avoiding relentless incandescent and fluorescent illumination systems. Artificial light, like artificial heat and cold, provides increased human convenience and comfort. Like other climate controls, electrically activated illumination systems are intimately involved with the economics of our modern technological states. That is, light as well as heat helps to condition human achievement and worker productivity. UVT (ultraviolet-transmitting) material is broadly marketed for installation as windows in all forms of human shelters and enclosures, and the same material is readily obtainable from optical firms and opticians making corrective "glasses." Examination of promotional literature distributed by manufacturers and marketers of conventional tinted dark glasses reveals that, while evidence is provided to remind readers of the possible harm of excessive exposure to ultraviolet radiation and "glare," these pamphlets and booklets are quite devoid of reference to the healthful benefits of ultraviolet presumed by medical specialists and researchers to be necessary for the promotion of normal, natural body weather.

# 4

# Climate, Weather, and Sexuality

**F**ertility and sexual functions in animals and man appear closely related to the combustion level the climate permits or encourages. It appears likely that the pituitary and adrenal glands, in affective relationship with metabolic processes, and controlling gonadal activities, respond promptly if the ease of body heat loss suddenly changes. In hot weather body heat loss is difficult; combustion processes are reduced, as is endocrine activity and, secondarily, the secretions of the sex glands. Is a change in sexual functioning a primary result of external environmental change or a secondary response to changes in the general metabolic level and glandular activity? No simple, final answer can be given, for human sexual activity among humans (especially males) is conditioned by an extraordinary range of cultural conditioners, rituals, traditions, expectations, and artificial stimuli, as well. More than one anthropologist or sexual therapist has observed that among males sex might well be considered about 90 percent mental. Nevertheless, it has been known for many centuries and provable since the last five decades that climate and weather affect human sexual responses.

## NATURAL WEATHER AND SEXUAL RESPONSES

### Climate and Sexual Maturity

One of man's best-preserved myths is that tropical girls mature earlier than temperate girls. Scientifically speaking, this is about on the same level of accuracy as the popular belief that redheads are supersexy or that blondes have more fun than brunettes. The myth of early-blooming tropical girls is most likely based on careless observations made by men more interested in sex than in science. All the data indicates the reverse condition to be true. Body development and growth is markedly retarded by tropical climates. Physically, the average tropical girl aged fifteen looks like a twelve-year-old girl born and raised in a cool region. Among many subtropical and tropical peoples, marriage follows immediately after first menstruation. Eighteenth- and nineteenth-century explorers, colonizers, and missionaries encountering substantial numbers of sixteen-year-old mothers may have assumed that sexual maturity began much earlier. Pioneer studies, like Margaret Mead's *Coming of Age in Samoa*, explicated the nature of early adolescent sexual training. Victorian man was scandalized and fascinated by the (to him) uninhibited enthusiasm tropical peoples exhibited for sexual intercourse. A variety of initiation rituals are blatantly erotic in all cultures. The merchant mariner and the missionary were struck by the overt and apparently casual sexiness of tropical peoples. The forthright and objective research of Richard Burton, the mid-Victorian explorer, was considered prurient and some of his work was suppressed or destroyed by his wife as pornography.

Legends of nubile girls waiting beneath the sheltering palms have been traced back as far as the writing of Hippocrates. In prehistoric times, when the polar icecap covered the North American continent south to Cincinnati, optimal conditions for human fertility and reproduction existed in what are now the planet's subtropical and tropical zones. As the earth warmed, these conditions shifted toward both poles and man moved after. Based on modern evidence, it seems accurate to state that nowhere do women mature so early as they do now in the center of North America and in west central Europe. The mean age for menarche in the American Middle West was thirteen years in 1935. The tendency continues, with the mean age dropping slightly. Throughout the tropics, women typically menstruated a full two years later, at about age fifteen.

Malnutrition delays the onset of the menses and so does a climate of long numbing cold, as in Finland or northern Russia.

Nutrition and climate are closely coordinated today, despite enormously improved rates of transportation and systems of food storage. Extreme climatic conditions limit the types of plants and animals adapted for survival. In climates too hot or too cold food is scanty, diet limited, and growth to maturity retarded. Generally speaking, stormy, energizing climates with abundant weather changes promote optimum conditions for sex as well as other significant activities.

When we consider the contemporary situation, with the increasingly artificial climates of modern urban areas, we discover that city girls tend to mature about one-half year earlier than rural girls. This may be due to the effects of prolonged and sustained cooling systems, the fact that the modern "heat-island" megalopolis ameliorates the frigid winter months, and/or the emotionally stimulating pace of city life.

First menstruation and the onset of fertility do not follow in one-two sequence. Normally, there is a time lag which seems to vary, but within a pattern: the earlier a girl menstruates, the sooner she will become fertile. The rate of growth has accelerated to a point where it can now be said that the period of female childhood has shortened somewhat. Girls become women earlier, but do not grow physically after the second year of menstrual activity. The long bones harden and the pelvic girdle spreads, but it is not uncommon for girls to carry their "baby fat" into their twenties, along with pubescent skin conditions, such as acne.

All this physical activity does not mean that North American women are sexier (which is behavioral), but rather that they respond physically to optimum nutrition, plus the stimulation of a temperate climate. Precocious sexual awakening and activity is very likely due to cultural stimuli from movies, television, and popular music, which have all become increasingly explicit and graphic in recent decades. It still remains a cultural tradition for the women of northern regions of the United States to marry somewhat later than southern belles. Northern girls may be fertile earlier, but southern women have shown a tendency to get themselves fertilized before their cool-climate sisters, thus perpetuating another sex myth, the "hot-blooded" Georgia peach. Since the same pattern of earlier menses and earlier fertility holds true for northern black women as well as white, it is a biological law, not a racial condition. The primary social concern now seems to have stabilized around the issue of birth control, family planning, and contraceptive systems. The effect of the North American climate, together with a growth-promoting diet, has been to produce a very large number of fertile women well below the age traditionally acceptable to parents as "marriageable"; many of them are sexually active.

## Climate and Conception

Male sex drive during the different seasons of the year tends to mimic the effects of climate. In Canada, for instance, the "conception curve" shows vitality peaking in midsummer but depressed in midwinter. Before Florida became almost totally air-conditioned, the sex situation was reversed. The long, humid summer months depressed sexual activity and the mild winter stimulated conception. Fertility seems to reach optimum conditions around sixty-five degrees Fahrenheit, declining in response to extremes of either heat or cold. The rate of conception can vary as much as 35 percent, under natural, normal conditions (Mills, 44–47).

Obviously, the situation has been considerably altered due to artificially stimulating climate controls and to artificial contraceptive devices utilized by unmarried and married women and men. It is probable that American sexual activity has increased somewhat, even as the population growth rate has dropped to zero or slightly above. The "baby boom" of the 1940s and 50s is over, and many towns and cities have the empty schools to prove it. It has become possible and to some degree more permissible for more people to have more sex, without undesired pregnancy resulting. The old poetic association of love and springtime still holds true, although our technology has effectively eliminated sexually depressing extremes of heat, humidity, and cold. To some real degree, although never measured, the automobile promotes sexual activity. Young men and women can obtain hours of privacy and rudimentary convenience inside parked cars, although it can be assumed that places to park those cars are not so easy to find, as our cities sprawl across the countryside, obliterating discreet country roads and lovers' lanes. Interested anthropologists have observed that contemporary dance fashions, while emphasizing pelvic gyrations, prohibit touching; so they look more arousing than they really are. Compared to the youth of other nations, American boys and girls honor social taboos and prohibitions, limiting their physical contacts in public to holding hands and strolling with arms around each other. Public kissing of Parisian enthusiasm is almost never observed.

Back in the late 1920s, when legal prostitution flourished in

Japan, the conception rate among Japanese women zoomed to annual peaks from mid-March into June. Then, as the summer settled into three months of hot, humid weather, the rate of conceptions plummeted, rising in a gentle slope up until the crescendo of the succeeding cherry blossom season. At this time, each house of prostitution was required to report its number of clients for each twenty-four-hour period. There was no comparable decline of male visitors, with client rates remaining quite stable, despite the summer discomfort. The only conclusion that researchers could reasonably draw was that Japanese males had intercourse at about the same rate with prostitutes year-round. The excessive heat and humidity must, therefore, have caused a drop in physiological fertility among Japanese women (Mills, 49–51).

The climate of temperate zones certainly accounts for the habit of the June marriage, although there are other, cultural conditioners as well—high school graduation times, for instance. Temperate-zone humans marry in large numbers in the autumn, also. While mid-summer conception is still common among newlyweds, no late-fall peak follows the second most common mating period. Despite the widespread use of both air conditioners and contraceptive devices, which might seem to offset each other, seasonal fluctuations in conception persist in the temperate zones and reflect real changes in human fertility, rather than variations in the marriage rate or frequency of intercourse, legal or illicit.

### The Natural Method of Birth Control

With the exception of those days of active menstruation, women can have intercourse, but their ovulation rhythm is normally such that conception is possible only for about four days out of twenty-eight, an approximate lunar month. This fact, widely publicized in recent decades, permits both a natural form of birth control for couples who wish to avoid conception by the female (and choose not to employ any contraceptive device or drug) and provides peak fertility information for couples eager to have children. In the first instance, the couple refrains from intercourse on the peak fertility days of the woman's cycle; in the second case, those days are preferred for intercourse as most likely to achieve insemination.

### Predetermining the Sex of Children

Predetermination of the sex of a child is claimed with accuracy over 90 percent by Czechoslovakian medical scientist Eugen Jonas.

His method derives from knowing the position of the moon in the sky at the time of conception. According to ancient astrologers, each of the zodiac signs has a sex. When the moon is in a male zone, intercourse which causes conception will produce a male child. In this way, couples aware of lunar phases and positions can determine, through intercourse, the sex of their offspring. According to Jonas, his calculations for 8,000 Czech women who wanted to bear male children provided them with the information that made this possible in 95 cases out of 100. Studies on methods of artificial insemination revealed that a weak electric current passed through a sample of semen tends to separate female from male spermatazoa. Since the moon is known to create alterations in the magnetic field of the earth, it is logical to believe that a kind of sorting process is made possible for predetermination of the sex of children yet unborn (Watson, 63).

### Best Months to be Born

The work of Jonas in his clinic at Bratislava is based on an extremely short cycle or rhythm, only two hours in length. Longer cycles appear involved in childbirth. For example, in the northern hemisphere, more children are born during the months of May and June than in November and December. This would seem to correspond to annual August vacation time for the parents. Curiously, children born in the month of May are heavier at birth by about two grams than infants born at any other month of the year. This correlation between weight and time of conception appears to depend on seasonal production of hormones involved with pregnancy and not lunar influences. In the southern hemisphere, the situation is reversed, with more robust children born in the period from December to February, the midsummer months "down under."

Some evidence now exists suggesting that there may be "best" months to be born in, and that longevity and intelligence are possibly affected by hormonal states during prenatal life. While long life depends on a number of cultural factors such as income, nutrition, and medical care, it appears that children born in New England in the month of March are likely to live four years longer, on the average, than children born in the same area, but during any other month of the year. Huntington's book, *Season of Birth: Its Relation to Human Abilities*, was based on the study of 17,000 New York schoolchildren. According to the study, those boys and girls born in May scored better on standardized IQ tests than those born at any other time of the year. Huntington's conclusions were based on data compiled in the late 1930s and never very widely accepted, in part because of skepticism concerning the validity of standardized tests in general and partly because he appears to be on the "wrong" side of the nature versus nurture controversy that lies beneath twentieth-century practices of child-rearing and educational methodologies. It is felt to be un-American to suggest that nature predetermines the achievement of children. Information that does not correspond to myth or need is regularly disregarded and its proponents sometimes subjected to unwarranted abuse.

### Sexual Orientation of the Unborn Child

The Society for the Scientific Study of Sex is headed by John Money, director of the psychohormonal research unit at the medical school of Johns Hopkins University. Money, in recent trial testimony, testified that, in his view, human sexual functioning is predetermined by physiological factors: "Once the die is cast hormonally, it cannot be reversed." Does this mean that natural (and, these days, artificial) environmental stimuli and hormonal responses during the mother's pregnancy permanently fix the development of sexual orientation? Apparently so, since Money earlier stated his belief that "prenatal hormones can predispose bi- or homosexual development." While Money allows for some degree of gender identification training and reinforcement through the long process of growth from infancy through adolescence, he has stated that "by adulthood, we don't have the potential any longer to be other than what we by then are—homosexual, bisexual or heterosexual." (*New York Times Magazine*, 9 November 1975, p. 60.)

This emphasis on physiological predetermination appears to be a new level of trust in what has been known or thought but forgotten. North Americans have been taught to believe that each human contains within himself the will and energy to improve, alter, and change. We have been fond of all sorts of "self-improvement" schemes, courses, and therapies, convinced that both males and females can "grow" into more fruitful and self-fulfilling utilization of individual physical and mental resources. Recently, the stern facts of environmental limitation have borne down hard upon us like a weight squeezing out some of our national romanticism. We are beginning to pass from suspicion to acceptance of scientific data that challenges rather than supports our generally optimistic view of life conditions. Investigations have now pushed past the domain of the sociologist and his processes of "acculturation" to the deeper, secret springs of health and human functioning within.

## Natural Light and Sexuality

Such an investigation into human sexual behavior and the newer field of psychohormonal responses mediated by the environment rather than by cultural training began with consideration of birds and their migratory and mating patterns. A change in light, alone, slows or speeds cycles of fat deposits and pre- and postmating responses, including the loss and regrowth of feathers. Birds acclimated by artificial light to the season of autumn, flew "south" when released in a planetarium simulating a spring sky. The actual month was May. The impact of light, alone, had altered physical responses by about six months (Luce, 123).

Why is it that environmental conditions of light in the spring make animals, including humans, sexier? Dr. Joseph Meites of Michigan State University explains the phenomenon this way: "In spring a young squirrel's fancy turns because the days are getting longer, and exposure to longer light periods sets off a chain-reaction involving the brain and pituitary gland, resulting in releases of hormones that affect sex hormone levels and in turn cause the sex glands to enlarge." His experiments confirmed the impact of light as stimulating the estrogen secretion of ovaries and male sperm production in smaller mammals. Cycles of light rather than intensity seem important, too. Like other animals, humans live within the basic light-dark rhythm of the rotating earth. All things considered, then, it seems fair to say that there is a mating season for humans which approximates that of other animals and for about the same physiological reasons. Psychologically, human sexuality is extremely complex, and seasonal influence may be more indirect. Light stimulates sex hormones at a time when warmer outdoor temperatures permit humans to wear less clothing. Unwrapped women appear to be more receptive to sex. Not only is there more light, but there is more for environmentally stimulated males to see when they look. Girl-watching is a male springtime activity. Scattered evidence exists which suggests that many women find the flattering attentions of males to be mildly stimulating, providing that a sense of decorum is maintained by silence.

Physiological cycles and responses, then, are regulated by the nervous system in its reaction to alternating light and darkness. Is i possible to isolate the center of human sexual responses through biochemical alterations conditioned by environmental light? Researchers now believe that the pineal gland is the major mediator of the relationship between light and sexual functioning.

### Secretions of the Light-sensitive Pineal Gland

The human pineal gland is a tiny structure embedded deep between the two hemispheres of the brain. Shaped like a pinecone, this gland typically protrudes from the skulls of lizards, covered with a thin layer of protective skin. In other animals, too, the pineal is larger in relation to brain mass than it is in man. It seems to be a sort of vestigial organ, perpetuated by heredity, but grown dwarfish over thousands of centuries, like the little toe on human feet. Yet much of our present knowledge about the pineal indicates that it plays a significant role in biochemical rhythms relating to environmental changes and impacts. Melatonin, a complex molecule of the same chemical family that is central to the transactions of the brain in mood swings when the human is awake and in the strange processes of sleep, exists in the tissue of the pineal gland. Moreover, a highly specialized enzyme that breaks down other molecules, transforming them into melatonin, is found *only* in the pineal gland. If pineal gland tissue was destroyed in infant rats, the animals attempted to copulate at abnormally early ages. In humans, disturbed pineal function was even more grotesque, with kindergarten males capable of adult sexual functions. Through melatonin secreted by the pineal gland sexuality appeared to be regulated, speeding up or slowing down, but primarily the latter.

Animals raised under constant light tend to produce more melatonin than those existing in darkness. However, experiments have assumed that incandescent bulbs or fluorescent tubes are acceptable as light sources, without consideration of the fact that each system transmits only a limited form of visible light and no ultraviolet. That is, these experiments appear based on the belief that all light is the same: visible, identical in effect, regardless of source, with intensity and duration more significant than wavelength. How valuable can these results be, when it is known that *natural* sunlight affects the development of the pineal gland itself? John Ott's experiments indicate that wavelength *is* important. Quite recently, Japanese researchers were able to prove that the pineal gland responds to different wavelengths of visible light; this suggests that the neuroendocrine system responds similarly. The fact that these reactions are described as "color sensitive" indicates that the researchers involved still believe in the effects of visible light, that is less than 1 percent of the total spectrum, and persist in believing that natural and artificial light are essentially the same, when they are vastly different. Quite possibly, all that can be learned, given these biases, has already been discovered: that pineal secretions fluctuate in daily rhythm synchronized by periods of light and dark.

A close relative of adrenaline, called norepinephrine, is stored in tiny cell-sacs in the nerve endings of the human body. The pineal gland is rich in this substance. The known sensitivity of the nerve-gland relationship to light might suggest that norepinephrine is part of the human alarm and excitement system. Like other secretions, norepinephrine shows a rising and falling rate influenced by light and dark—that is, by the wavelength of light—plus intensity and duration of light. This substance is crucial to health-sustaining functions such as body temperature, brain temperature, and the daily rise and decline of adrenaline hormones and is considered to be a "drive" substance, the intermediary of basic life functions: waking, alertness, hunger, vitality, sex arousal and function, drowsiness and sleep (Luce, 127).

Obviously, any human would suffer major disorientation, disfunction, and death without an internal management and drive system to synchronize and regulate the basic life functions in relationship with the natural environment. Conversely, dramatic and prolonged manipulation of the environment affects the pineal gland and its secretions, and so affects the sympathetic nervous system and other glands.

Light is not incidental. Light is critical. Male hamsters, notoriously sexy, when deprived of light suffer shrinkage of their gonads to one-quarter normal size with accompanying depressed sexual activity. Eskimo women in the Arctic often do not menstruate during the winter. Once accepted as a response to numbing cold, it seems more likely to be the result of deprivation of wavelengths of natural sunlight (Mills, 51).

Light appears to be as potent as a drug, although medical science has been indifferent to its probable usefulness in both preventive and curative capacities. In an increasingly artificial environment, humans have acquired new health habits, many of them damaging. Man simply assumes that he switches light on and off. The facts indicate that the reverse is true: light switches man on and off. From the prenatal hormones through the rate of maturation of the pineal gland in newborn infants, light affects us all from the first instant of conception. Light triggering the rhythmic rise and fall of hormone secretions, light impinging on the entire neuroendocrine system, light as part of the emergency warning system—all indicate the critical importance of solar irradiation.

### The Impacts of Invisible Natural Light

Although not yet proved, the impacts of invisible natural light appear to be equally, if not more significant than the tiny percentage of light humans are able to perceive. Color sensitivity and responses are primarily if not totally cultural. (What we call "red" is so only because that is the name English-speaking people have agreed that reflection shall be called. We could have called that reflection "blue" or "xyz" and it would *look* the same. Along with naming, we have assigned the symbolic significances of colors: red for embarrassment or anger, white for purity or fear, black for death, blue for the Virgin Mary, and so forth.) Wavelength responses and reactions are physiological and totally *un*learned. Precisely because humans perceive what they call colors and because their cultures have come to give certain colors certain significance, their habits of thinking about light are seriously inhibited. It is quite likely, after all, that given photoreceptor mechanisms that respond to wavelength and many body cells, tissues, and organs that respond to invisible irradiations (including infrared and X-rays), human color perceptions are irrelevant to human health, well-being, and sexual function. Dogs, among other animals, do not perceive color. The bull in the ring does not "see red" and charge the magenta cape of the Spanish *torero*, but attacks movement within his territory, quite a different set of concepts altogether. Color perception and emotional responses, created by language and acculturation, may make life more psychologically enjoyable, but could be quite gratuitous, a kind of creative "freebie" thrown in with more important and more affective impacts of light that modify and moderate human body weather.

## ARTIFICIAL WEATHER AND SEXUAL RESPONSES

Much that has already been noted about human sexuality as responding to climate, weather, and light has included references to the increasing use of machinery or electrical energy to maintain conditions known to be conducive to human productivity. To a real degree, the techniques of manipulating heat, cold, humidity, and light have affected human reproductivity as well, at a time when heightened levels of awareness and permissiveness encourage or tolerate methods of population control, including mechanical and pharmaceutical contraceptives. The extremes of control, abortion and euthanasia, causes disturbed responses from men and women and not, by any means, on religious grounds alone. It is true that humans have tended to equate sexuality, the creation of life, and death, the termination of life, with religion more than they have the conditions of environment. As man over the centuries has moved to a position of increased comfort and convenience, he has been able to dispense with his earlier preoccupation with natural climate, weather, and light. As modern man has become less subject to seasonal disasters like flood and famine, his sexual and fertility rituals have almost disappeared. The religions of today are primarily intellectual rather than physical and seek to govern human behavior, including sexual behavior, by ethical standards. Ancient man prayed that his copulations would prove fertile. Modern man prays that his tendencies in the sexual area will not be held sinful and/or socially inappropriate. We do not think of Easter as the beginning of our rutting season and have dismantled or desexed those few pagan sex ceremonies that have survived. While not entirely climate- or weather-proof, human sexuality seems to have little relationship to the natural environment out of which man has evolved, but an increasingly disturbing relationship to the impacts of the cultures he has created.

Since warm, well-fed humans abound in North America, it can be said that almost nobody's sex life is dominated by the climate, except for annual fertility peaks, which are truly biological, operating with nondiscriminate effect on all women regardless of race or social class. Extreme heat and humidity depress sexual activity, and it is assumed that air conditioning in homes, schools, and automobiles has some statistically unverifiable effect on North American sexual activity, while social permissiveness and widely distributed contraceptive devices maintain an offsetting level of population growth.

**The Sexual Revolution**

North Americans have become significantly less inhibited about their own sexual functioning, to the degree that sociologists and anthropologists note a new, more permissive social attitude. All the factors contributing to freer use of taboo words, greater degrees of sexual initiative among younger women, and displays of human nudity and explicit sex acts in the legitimate theater and on movie

*119*

and home television screens appear to add up to cultural changes that some have called "the sexual revolution." Doctors and social workers point out the astonishing rise in the rate of venereal disease among all classes of North American youth. Neither increased social acceptance of sexuality nor the infection rate attributed to frequent, casual intercourse can be traced to the furnace in the basement or the air conditioner in the bedroom in a cause-effect relationship. Virginity is not regulated by thermostat, nor adultery by an electrical switch.

The new permissive sexual "climate" then is an alteration of cultural and social attitudes, not a significant change in natural environment and only by indirect extension traceable to the mechanical devices manufactured to raise the standard of human comfort. After all, Victorian Americans enjoyed much more central heating than their grandparents; yet the period in which they lived was one of sexual repression, not permissiveness.

What modern man tends to think of as sexual functioning is copulation technique (preferably illustrated), with some advice or therapy for improved frequency and rate of orgasmic satisfaction. Neither sexual therapy nor the "climate" of culture belongs within the pages of a book seeking to explicate body weather. Moreover, the impacts of increased levels of comfort have never been analyzed. The most authoritative studies deal primarily with the psychology of sexual response and secondarily provide information on the physiology of sexual excitement and fulfillment. Neither the early studies by Kinsey or any later work considers the season or weather as factors in human sexual functioning. Can it be, then, that artificial climate control and weather manipulation is entirely irrelevant to human sexual responses? No, but much that can and will be said below proceeds from common sense and generalized observations. The tendency of a modern technology to standardize the culture containing it permits some few conclusions.

### Comfort Levels and Sexual Behavior

We have seen throughout these pages that weather, defined as the short-term sum of a dozen environmental conditions, does affect humans promptly, regularly, and significantly. Abrupt, sharp change, typical of the passage of storm fronts through a region, measurably affects human metabolism and may be considered to predispose human beings to a variety of diseases. The most stimulating weather conditions in the world are to be found in the northern central region of the United States, within the V-shaped trough in the pattern of storms passing across the continent from west to east. Individuals respond to the stimulation of weather in known and predictable ways, with variation due to sex, age, body type, weight, geographical area, and elevation above sea level. The point at which stimulation becomes stress—with resulting direct and indirect influences upon organs, systems, tissues, and cells—has been determined approximately, but again the range of human responses is quite broad. Human adaptability is a marked characteristic of the species and people quickly learn to react to weather in ways which support or sustain thermodynamics typical of mammals in general.

Women generally appear capable of enduring heat at levels that men find uncomfortable. Even well-motivated males exhibit a deterioration of mental performance under hot conditions and tend to sweat more profusely. Women complain of discomfort from cold, and their physical and mental responses indicate decreased activity when the temperature of the air around them falls to levels supported by males without discomfort.

Since artificial weather is engineered for human convenience and comfort and tends to eliminate the stressful impacts of storms, it would appear to permit human sexual activity at a relatively standard rate, regardless of seasonal change. Both men and women seek warmth and privacy as primary conditions for sexual intercourse. Physical discomfort and accompanying mental distress discourage sexual intimacy, and the surroundings acceptable for many forms of work or recreation inhibit sexual activity. The preferred site for sexual intercourse is the bedroom, and the typical time is after dark, but these factors of place and time are learned as part of the total acculturation of the individual. So, too, are preferred days of the week. It is likely that Saturday night could be established statistically as the time of greatest sexual activity. Certainly the midwinter holidays, a span of relaxed inhibitions, and early summer, habitual vacation time, encourage increased sexual activity, but here, again, the influence of the containing culture is assumed to act as a conditioner greater than any stimulus derived from local manipulation of weather.

Physical confinement among members of the same sex does appear to have a sexually depressing effect upon women, especially younger women experiencing military service, prison, hospitalization, or single-sex schooling. Menstruation may become irregular, and the period of menses shorter; sometimes menstruation ceases altogether. For such women, vacation, leave, or release seems to

*121*

have a markedly exciting effect, lowering inhibition and raising readiness for sexual activity. Although no studies have been reported, the physiology of males does not appear to be affected in a comparable manner, although periodic deprivation may cause emotional strain.

As we have seen, human fertility follows annual cycles and artificial control of climate and weather appears to have no significant effect on conception, although it may be assumed that optimum conditions of convenience and comfort promote sexual intercourse at the " normal" frequency rate. However, no agreement exists among researchers as to what rate is normal or even fairly typical. A very considerable number of factors such as general state of health, level of fatigue, mood, surroundings, desirability of partner, and highly individualized psychological states of being probably will prevent the establishment of a mean rate of frequency for males or females. What is "normal" given the total body weather of a healthy and attractive woman in her mid-twenties might be more frequent, less frequent, or about the same number of intercourse experiences as the same subject later in life, as another subject of the same age group, or not really comparable at all. This is likely true of males, as well. So many variables and unknowns are involved that it seems most accurate to state that the frequency of human sexual intercourse varies randomly. Controlled conditions simply do not exist.

### The Blackout of 1965

Only once in recent human history has a freak of artificial weather triggered a measurable response of human sexual activity. In November of 1965, a massive power failure caused a blackout in the northeastern United States. Millions lost light and heat, the services of electric kitchens, and electric-powered modes of transportation: elevators, escalators, and subways. Workers were trapped in high-rise office buildings and inside elevator cars. Unknown and uncounted casual encounters between men and women were prolonged through the early evening into the early morning of the following day. What might have been a catastrophic situation resulting from widespread panic appears to have been accepted as a kind of artificial holiday. The weather was typically cold and mechanical heating systems dependent upon electricity were unable to function. For one evening, modern human beings were flung back in time to a rough approximation of life conditions standard in the almost forgotten past. Emergency radio networks continued to function, but television transmission ceased and other forms of spectator recreation such as the movies or legitimate theater were unavailable. Cooked food was available only to those persons with gas or camping stoves, chafing dishes, or the like. Warmth and light was limited to those homes and apartments equipped with one or more fireplaces and oil lamps or candles. Untold numbers of spouses were separated, and extraordinary physical exploits were required for reunion. A sort of "survivor spirit" seems to have possessed many millions in the course of this unexpected change in artificial weather. Loss of light and loss of heat were the most critical experiences. Deprived of convenience and comfort, isolated and unobservable, denied the standard diversions that modern urban dwellers accept as a matter of course, millions of men and women simply went to bed.

### *"Blackout Babies"*

The results were an astonishing number of births, legitimate and illegitimate, in late July and early August of 1966. "Blackout babies" were born in numbers astronomically above the norms for midsummer. Never before nor since have men and women engaged in sexual intercourse in such numbers within a given time period. Immediate and intimate causes can be assumed to have varied: the need for physical warmth, the opportunity to satisfy suppressed desires for illicit sexual union, recreational sex excited by a sort of carnival atmosphere and mood, conscious or unconscious fear of extinction, intercourse as a substitute for other forms of recreation, and release of psychological tensions. The primary cause of this extraordinary binge of human sexual behavior was obviously the sudden change in artificial weather—the abrupt, unanticipated loss of control over internal heat and light within urban and suburban shelters during the early winter season within a temperate zone.

Would repeated instances cause a comparable sexual response? Since a decade has passed and the phenomenon of the "blackout baby" has disappeared except as a kind of "in" joke among parents of the 1966 crop and the members of the medical profession providing obstetrical and nursing services, the tendency is to think "yes," with slightly less astounding birth rates nine months following, due to more widespread and regular use of contraceptive methods. At least such a response would seem probable, based on the scattered evidence combined with a common-sense awareness that comparable conditions tend to produce comparable results. Since humans habituate so readily, a significant number of massive power failures would probably have a diminishing effect on sexual response. That is, the more often urban blackouts occurred, the less attention both men and women would give them. The holiday mood would dissipate, and the loss of control over artificial weather would become readily acceptable as another inescapable nuisance of urban life. The only evidence that can be offered is sociological, not biochemical or medical-obstetrical. Citizens inhabiting urban centers showed a remarkable capacity to adapt to massive air raids during World War II. Early terror, excitement, and loss of emotional inhibitions were replaced by a stoic acceptance of bombing attack.

Executives responsible for the maintenance of the Northeast power grid have repeatedly declared that the massive blackout of the urbanized region cannot happen again. Once, by error or malfunction, but not twice. Major alterations in the vast electrical complex were made. Since the nature of all physical life is change and not stasis, and the second law of thermodynamics explicates the tendency of all things to decline in efficiency and finally to fail or cease functioning altogether and the human ability to control that which is artificial is not absolute, it is difficult to believe that another unanticipated, widespread, and prolonged collapse of artificial weather will never happen. It is, no doubt, extremely unlikely. Overall, the experience of those dark and cold hours of November, 1965 was comic rather than tragic. No seizure of terror gripped the urban centers most affected. Police records and insurance forms showed a peak of minor traffic accidents and hospitals handled exceptional numbers of victims of falls and burns, plus a disquieting increase of heart attack victims, felled by unusual physical exertion, as they labored up flights of stairs ten, twenty, and thirty stories above street level. The incidence of violent crime was about as usual and reported looting was unexpectedly low.

The major human response to this night-long loss of control over artificial weather was a sexual response, a kind of procreative promiscuity. Since the experience was unique, little meaning can be derived from it. It does not argue, for example, that humans today are more or less sexually active than their ancestors. The record simply states that when the lights go off and the heat in homes and buildings declines below the level of customary comfort, human beings—temporarily excited, bored, cold, or anxious—will go to bed with spouses, acquaintances, or comparative strangers if able to do so. Once there, many will engage in sexual intercourse. Given the known propensity for conception among healthy women of child-bearing ages, an extraordinary number will become pregnant and give birth approximately nine months later. The blackout of 1965 may demonstrate, to an optimist, desirably typical human response to the unexpected and possibly life-threatening. A pessimist, considering the same experience, might comment on the lack of human imagination. What else was there to do?

# 5

# Wind, Noise,
# and Irradiation

Initially, it may not be easy to understand why or how three very different physical facts can be gathered for consideration. Wind and vibration might be construed to have indirect effects on human physical and mental well-being, but certainly some forms of irradiation directly affect the growth of certain kinds of cells. Movement of air is obviously involved with sensations, touch in the case of wind and hearing in the case of air-transmitted vibration, the most common form. Irradiations from chemical substances, electronic devices, or the nearer stars pass through the air, but are not transmitted in the same manner as noise, music, or human speech. The nature of human response, also, is very different. Wind and vibration can be pleasant or distressing experiences, but the most powerful of irradiations, the X rays, cannot be felt at all. The effect of irradiations on the human body may be profound and enduring; the passage of a spring breeze is mild, transitory, and casual. The fact that both phenomena are invisible seems no more than coincidental.

For the purpose of analyzing how these life conditions affect human body weather, we are assuming a category: intimacy. Obviously, in the abstract and highly specific areas of the several sciences, the word "intimacy" is without meaning. Perhaps a biologist might employ the word to describe certain types of behavior, even as a synonym or substitute for "density" or "crowding." The word appears in scientific considerations of human sexuality, erotic foreplay, emotional affinities, and so on. Here, in consideration of the impacts of environment on human body weather, the word is intended to limit consideration of responses to the individual, not the group, and at the same time to communicate some concepts of subtle and sometimes strange emotional responses associated with private physical experiences. We use the words "intimacy" and "intimate," then, in an extrascientific way and do not intend them to be quantitatively precise, but humanistic and suggestive, as they might be applied to the very brief and very old anonymous poem quoted below:

> O, Western wind, when wilt thou blow,
> That the small rain down shall rain?
> Christ! That my love were in my arms,
> And I in my bed again.

Sometimes printed as it may originally have been written, in two long lines, the strange piece of verse has puzzled and intrigued critics and interpreters. A good deal has been written about the poem, out of all proportion to the twenty-eight words that comprise its total statement. It is, evidently, an "intimate" poem. The speaker, whom most students assume or "know" to be male, is not so much talking to the wind, as using the wind as a means of expressing what is on his mind: an excruciating sense of lonely longing and sexual frustration. It has been argued that the man is in England, separated from his love by the Irish Sea. The western wind is seasonal, generally from that direction in the spring. Ireland and England both get a good deal of rain, but "small" rain falls in the spring. In the poem, "small rain" does not refer to inches of precipitation, but rather describes the delicate, feather-soft rain just barely more than mist for which the Spanish have a lovely descriptive phrase, *dedos de los angeles*, or "angels' fingers." Some readers believe the man's choice of words is more Irish than English, suggesting he is in exile or that he learned the phrase from his lady and that the gentle caress of the rain recalls her to his mind. Perhaps one might even assume that the girl is herself small and gentle. At any rate, there is no question of the lover's state of mind in the last two lines. A single, passionate cry. What he wants is so simple, so masculine, and so very human that untold numbers of readers are moved to sympathy. The cadence or meter of the lines is somehow both commonplace, the stuff of everyday speech, and the words so simple that they combine for us in a whole greater than the sum of its apparent parts. It is a great love poem, as well as serving here as an exemplar of our category of intimate impacts.

## THE DISTRESSING IMPACT OF WIND

Air in motion, flowing like invisible water, can be rather complex as a fact of the physical environment. Insofar as it touches an individual, it has significance for body-weather states. Air transmits information and transports substances likely to affect human well-being. Odors, especially strong or pungent smells like that of burned wood, are wind-transmittable. Yeasts, bacilli, and other microorganisms are swirled over vast distances by the wind. Strong, steady wind powerful enough to lift inorganic particles can cause extreme human inconvenience and discomfort to the point of severe stress, as the passage below makes very clear (Cousteau, 125):

> A catastrophic week passed by. Every afternoon, the haboob, that violent storm of burning sand, beat down on the ship and prevented us from working. At about two o'clock, the sky above the western horizon would turn a reddish-gold and the sea would cease to live, its surface becoming absolutely motionless, seeming almost solid. The already stifling temperature became intolerable; our bodies ran with sweat and every movement was torture, aggravated by the rash of prickly heat with which we were all afflicted. Then the storm was on us and the howling wind raised little spouts of water that mingled with the sand and covered everything with a coating of yellowish, destructive mud. . . . As soon as it became possible to work again, we were forced to put in what seemed interminable hours of meticulous cleaning in order to protect our delicate and valuable equipment. Our eyes red and swollen, we moved about like automatons in a sandy, unbearable universe.

Certainly the author, Philippe, son of the world-renowned oceanographer, Jacques-Yves Cousteau, could have recorded this experience with a climatological wind rose and an index of particulate density correlated with wind speed, humidity index, ambient air temperature, and daily atmospheric pressure readings. But the intimacy of his personal experience of the haboob would vanish. As the passage stands written, we are able to share, vicariously, in his human *feelings*. For purely physiological reasons, Cousteau's wind, also blowing out of the west, causes him to feel that the passage of time is interminable, just as the unknown poet suffered the slow cycle of the year. One senses that both men, for different reasons, have red and swollen eyes and exist like automatons in environments totally different, but equally tormenting.

Human beings have little tolerance for wind. Speeds above twenty miles per hour become annoying, frustrating work and recreation, swirling up dust that irritates the membranes of the nose and throat and capable of causing acute discomfort to the eye. The human skin, buffeted by strong winds, transmits distress signals to the brain. Some primitive instinct causes us to feel uneasy, anxious, even prey to dread. The windstorm outside us creates an intimate response of physical and psychological discomfort.

When wind becomes the dominant feature of weather, as in the *mistral*, the *sirocco*, or the *haboob*, humans seem to become emotionally disoriented. This is no gentle breeze, soft as a caress or the touch of spiritual fingers, but a kind of torture, a flogging of the nerve-endings by an invisible, relentless force. Humans are well aware that vegetation is stunted and deformed by wind prevailing from a fixed quarter. Even when ground speed is less than gale force, which gives the individual good cause to be anxious for his physical safety, the intimate impact of wind seems to cause the human spirit to quail. We are as eager to get out of the wind as we are joyous in emotional response to the light touch of the spring breeze, which seems fickle, playful, and sensual. Modern man in his urban heat-islands has rather limited experiences of wind as pleasure-evoking or soothing, although waves of air pouring between the concrete and glass walls of the city canyons are the only force capable of "washing" health-damaging pollutants from city air.

## THE DISTRESSING IMPACT OF CALM

Humans do not typically experience pleasure from periods of calm, even in rural locations. Convection currents, as we have seen, aid in loss of body heat, a necessary condition for physical and emotional well-being during summer in temperate zones. The calm, we have learned, precedes the storm. Physiologically and psychologically, too, we respond to a rapid change in atmospheric pressure.

Our combustion rate alters and we can sense a slight increase in the effort needed to sustain existence. Extremely sensitive individuals endure distressing sensations of suffocation during periods of calm, when the air seems to envelop the body in an invisible sheet. On the other hand, if air temperature is low, even close to freezing on the Fahrenheit scale, motionless air appears to be more easily tolerated, especially so at night. The brilliant stars of a cloudless winter night combine with stimulating, even stressing cold to create internal feelings of exhilaration. The leaden sky of a windless winter day is emotionally depressing, as temperate-zone humans have learned to anticipate snow.

## THE WIND-CHILL FACTOR

About the first of November, radio and television weather forecasters provide listener-viewers with the wind-chill factor: the speed of air in motion at ground level combining with its temperature to increase the numbing and activity-depressing impact. The faster the wind blows, the colder it feels to us. This sort of information has a psychological effect as well. We are chilled emotionally, so to speak, as well as physiologically and tend to suffer with corresponding intensity, because we feel we should.

## HOW MEN AND WOMEN REACT TO WIND

To some degree, the intensity of human responses to wind appears instinctive and sexually differentiated, although no body of statistical information seems to exist which might provide factual evidence. The physical responses of the emergency alarm system in all mammals seem to cause immobilization of both the young and the females. Fear often causes fainting in women and children. The reason appears to be simple. Motionlessness or passivity is non-threatening behavior and likely, under the circumstances of a purely natural world, to improve the chances for survival. Animal or human predators may neglect the motionless female and her offspring. The male animal response is usually quite different: an instinctive outpouring of adrenal hormones and consequent mobilization of glucose reserves for immediate energy, combined with visible paling, the result of widespread constriction of the surface vascular system, a double protection minimizing bleeding from wounds and preparing the muscles for flight or combat.

Men seem to have instinctively stronger physiological and psychological responses to wind, which presumably have some survival function. Even casual observation permits a dramatic difference to be noted. Men and women wearing shirts, jackets, and pants do not usually behave in the same manner when experiencing a strong, buffeting wind. Males tend to face into it and squint, tilting or leaning against the uneven pressure, with the head tilted up and the facial muscles clenched in a combative grimace, a sort of ferocious smile. Men seem, to some degree, pleased by the challenge. A trouser-clad female, on the other hand, tends to hide her face or to avert it from strong gusts. This may be a culturally conditioned response, a sort of cosmetic flinch. Skirted females tend to turn completely around. Faced away from strong irregular winds, the woman's skirt is more manageable. A sense of modesty, an acculturated response, rather than physical preservation instincts seem to condition this about-face, although it has been plausibly suggested that female breasts are sensitive to cold (there being much more mass in mammalian tissue than in the flatter muscle slabs of the male chest, decorated with two rudimentary and practically useless nipples) and the nipples extremely so. Chill can shock nursing females to such a degree that milk-flow is seriously inhibited. If this is the case, then the faced-about posture of women is again life-preserving for nursing young.

Human males appear to exhibit greater restlessness when exposed to the intimate impact of wind, while human females tend to seek shelter. Males seem stimulated to muscular activity, a kind of nervous shifting and casting-about that could be controlled by the sympathetic nervous system as part of the emergency warning system programed into mammals. As males are known to be more easily discomforted by excessive heat than females, so they seem more easily excited by strong winds, even indoors, quite as if the sound of tossing trees or the sight of swiftly driven clouds triggers some instinctive alarm, creating unconscious behavior typical of caution or fear. Powerful winds, gusting and veering in direction, disperse even strong odors and disrupt the transmission of sound. It could be that even today, modern man inside the artificial shelter of his microclimates responds with deep-buried dread to those environmental conditions that enable a predator to steal dangerously close, undetected, or natural disaster to befall the man, his mate and cubs. For all our technology, certain specific conditions of the natural environment seem to cause spasms of aggressive or precautionary behavior, inbred from time immemorial, in the human male.

## VIBRATIONS, GOOD AND BAD

The human senses have developed highly specialized functions, but as the human brain enlarged, each of the senses became somewhat restricted in range. Human stereoscopic vision, ideal for depth perception and observation of objects moving in space, is combined with the ability to see a technicolored world. But we are able to see only 1 percent of the full spectrum of natural light, and eyes designed for hunting are poorly adapted for close-range work, such as the years of reading modern schooling requires. It is assumed that the human sense of smell was much more keen in prehistoric times, and that the men and women of 100,000 years ago lived in more intimate relationship with the odors of their environment. Humans who have pets are made aware regularly that the dog's senses of smell and hearing far exceed the same sense-receptors in man. Only when one sense is damaged or destroyed, does the human mechanism adapt, regaining to some degree the acuteness of another sense. Blind humans seem to relearn sharper hearing, becoming extremely sensitive to echoes which help them to locate large solid objects within spaces they can no longer see.

Vibration sensitivity appears to be important to humans, and this capacity is not limited to the sense of hearing, but includes the sense of touch. The extremities are especially acute, and the nerve endings of the hands and the feet are fine-tuned receptors of air- or earth-transmitted vibrations. Hundreds of thousands of other nerve endings buried beneath the surface of the skin pick up vibrations and flash information to the brain, where sense-messages are received, sorted, compared with information already stored in memory cells, and acted upon.

### Noise

The environment of man emits three kinds of vibrations with which humans interact in intimate relationships. First, a sort of rise-and-fall vibration, either of short duration or constant to the area, normally air-transmitted but in no regular or synchronic relationship with any other vibration or with itself. This is what we call "noise," and each human must learn to recognize several hundred which occur with some frequency within his environment. As a system of warning and reward, noise is obviously very important to human survival. Humans can learn rather quickly to anticipate noise and locate its approximate source. To some degree, then, we learn to "read" those vibrations characterized by the absence of regular time intervals that we call noise. Persons living within environments where noise emissions are largely nonmechanical possibly can hear a slightly larger range of vibrations than persons whose environments resound to mechanical noises. Modern man in an urban environment hears more noise in terms of volume, but measurably fewer *kinds* of noise than aboriginal man.

## Noise Pollution

As we have had occasion to note, human responses to extreme environmental conditions tend to be negative, measured in health terms. Too little noise is almost as unendurable as a sustained deafening racket. Any modern technology is very noisy and massive vibrations assault the human ears and skin. We not only hear "noise pollution," but feel it. So, too, with silence. These extremes are both stressors of human physiological and psychological responses. Too much prolonged racket actually damages the hearing mechanism and blunts brain response. Loud noises shock the human system, altering the insulin and glucose relationship, accelerating heartbeat rate, blood pressure, and respiration, and stressing the metabolic process. Response can range from panic and flight to a grim, dogged acceptance that becomes habitual, but never healthful. Stress is high at the beginning of a shift in a factory, for instance, but the workers respond with the general adaptation syndrome discussed in chapter 2. When humans are forced to endure environments they cannot escape, they are damaged to some degree both physically and psychologically. Serious sense-deprivation is a cruel and unusual punishment. Solitary confinement is a distressing torment. Generally speaking, when noise ceases to be information that the brain can make use of and becomes merely a condition of the environment, it may be considered to be a stressor capable of serious damage to the human body and mind. Rather like the intimate impact of wind, vibrations are not very easily tolerated. Humans are easily annoyed or distracted by noise and, just as they are affected by light they cannot see, men and women suffer from vibrations they cannot hear. One of the tyrannical assaults of the modern megalopolis on its inhabitants consists of its almost constant vibrations. The level of noise may rise and fall, but it never ceases. The very pavement on which the traffic rolls day and night quivers in response to motor vibrations. The rock from which high buildings rise trembles slightly, ceaselessly.

Human health responses to vibrations above or below the range of normal hearing include headache, insomnia, digestive upset, ulcers, cardiac strain, and perhaps other diseases. Human beings are engineered to "read" vibrations, but not to endure them.

## Music

Plant life is known to respond to vibration to the degree that sound-shocks and what we call noise stunt growth of some varieties. Geraniums, on the basis of one experiment cited in *The Secret Life of Plants*, seem to "prefer" the Brandenburg Concertos to rock and roll. What likely conditions plant responses are, first, the volume and intensity of music, and the fact that music is vibrations synchronized with intervals of time. Plants, like other life-forms, are time-contained and exhibit rather precise circadian rhythms and seasonal responses to light wavelengths.

Not all animals emit vibrations, although the vast majority make some sort of noise, often pitched and interrupted by silence. The noise may be a call, cry, chirp, or croak that warns others of its species, announces control within a food-gathering territory, or is associated with mating and reproduction. Mammals, the so-called higher species, are known to emit more (and more varied) vibrations than stridulating insects or songbirds. Dogs howl, yelp, "give tongue," or croon when they are pleased. Cats emit a sort of music, too, associated with their rather melodramatic love lives. Those mammals regarded as closer to man, the dolphins and the whales, are considered to be music makers. Long-playing records featuring whale songs have sold many thousands of copies. The melodies of these huge aquatic mammals are profoundly affecting to some humans. Whales sing in a surprising range, alter rhythm, and seem to appreciate harmony or at least be able to control pitch at will. The plaintive melodic songs of right whales vibrate through the ocean depths and can be heard up to 300 miles away by other whales. Whale songs are rather melancholy, often in a minor key, but clearly composed. They vary in length from a few seconds to several minutes; each whale seems to sing his own songs, and some evidence exists that the singer alters some of his songs with each season of mating, which suggests that the melodies of whales are comparable to the military marches and gentle ballads of man: they announce presence or warn other males and express longing for the opposite sex.

At its simplest, all music is vibration and distinguishable from what we call noise by controlled intervals of silence. A piece of music may be almost continuous vibrations or consist of up to 80 percent silence. Pitch, the up-and-downness of music, is also a characteristic of noise. The controlled, artificial manipulation of intervals of sounds and silences in one or more arrangements of time is central to the kind of vibration significant to the emotional life of man that we call music.

## The Stress of Musical Performance

The making of music is not an art alone, but work. Composition is math-based and performance is combustion-based, since it requires considerable amounts of energy. As a form of work, music is moderately stressing, since great precision is required, along with regular and prolonged repetition, and the allowable range of inaccuracy is very small indeed. Performers may be assumed to utilize the active stress hormone, norepinephrine, at levels approximating those of actresses, television performers, race car drivers, and public speakers. The pulse accelerates to about 150 heartbeats per minute, approximately twice the normal speed of cardiac labor (Carruthers, 70).

## How Music Affects the Listener

To a lesser degree, the human listener responds physiologically to that kind of vibration we call music. A good many learned responses are involved, of course, but very young children will mimic in motion the time rate and intervals of music they hear. Setting prior emotional associations to one side ("Listen, darling, they're playing our song!"), limited physical responses can be activated that are synchronized with performance. Respiration and heartbeat rates change in reaction to the compelling brass harmonies and pounding drums of a military march, and slow, melancholy melodies can effect metabolic changes in sensitive persons. Woodwind, string, brass, and percussion instruments provoke human emotional reactions, many of them learned, to be sure, but others that seem innate in man or associated with his instincts. Human physiological and psychological responses, which can be abrupt, acute, and prolonged by musical vibrations, powerfully affect male and female listeners. These responses are more strongly exhibited and felt by the listener when he is in the physical presence of the performers. Live music has an augmented intimate impact on man, since the vibrations are felt by the exposed skin as well as sensed through the ears. The "contact-high" of rock concert audiences is only slightly more affective than that experienced by audience members listening to a symphony. Opera may possibly be the strongest vibrator of the spectator's body and mind, since it is such a rich combination of simultaneous stimuli: instrumental and vocal performance; colorful costumes, lights, and sets; inner emotional tensions caused by the melodramatic incidents portrayed, and the extraordinarily complex blend of all the above. Performances by rock music groups are self-evidently debased opera: the units are there, but the arrangement emphasizes repetition of musical patterns and rhythms rather than variation and contrast. Voice amplification is electronic rather than the product of years of training and practice. Lights, stage activity, and very rudimentary dancing by costumed exhibitors are a parody of operatic performance on one hand and tribal ritual on the other.

Rock music, considered as a physical affector, rather than a cultural phenomenon, is quite powerful, therefore not insignificant. Unlike opera, during which the audience delays its joint response until the aria, scene, or act terminates, the rock concert audience responds in rough synchronization with the musicians.

We have used two forms of music to illustrate the power of musical vibrations to evoke human muscular, metabolic, and empathetic reactions. Perhaps, the intimate impacts can be better understood using the analogy of athletics. Humans react to some kinds of vibrations describable as music rather like a pole-vaulter. There is a short sprint acceleration, mild physical shock, abruptly soaring systems responses, and a rapid but harmless return to the original level. Other musical vibrations may be analogized to the mile runner. Human responses are warmup, gradual acceleration to best pace, stamina maintenance that draws on previously stored energy sources, and an adrenalized "kick" sprint to the finish at the level of exhaustion. In either case, although modern man often declines to notice his own physical and emotional responses to music, he is affected and can be stressed, willingly or not, by the kinds of musical sounds he can hear, feel, and make.

Finally, it is worth considering two well-known examples of human physical and emotional response to the intimate impacts of musical vibrations. These examples are political and economic. The justification for their inclusion here is simple: man is a political and economic animal in both the physical and the psychological senses.

## Wind, Noise, and Irradiation

Few organizations in man's history have so skillfully manipulated citizen constituencies as did the National Socialists in Germany during the 1930s. One of their most effective methods was the carefully staged political rally, a set show-piece arranged to make maximum use of vibrations: noise, music, and speech. The purpose was to evoke and exploit loyalty, to convert isolated skeptics into enthusiastic supporters. Huge crowds, already affective as noise, were synchronized by martial music—strident, prideful, and hypnotically aggressive. Speech, the third form of vibration affector, was reduced to intervaled chanting in response to the national leader, Adolf Hitler. The concepts of timing, mass, cadence, volume, and intensity of sound were systematized to exert control over the people of Germany.

Environmentalists are often thought of as outdoors people. Many, however, employ their skills at manipulating interior spaces and thus indirectly the humans those spaces contain. Again, the use of music is of great significance, this time in both ends of the economy: production and consumption. "Canned" music is known to improve worker production and to damp feelings of alienation among workers simultaneously, regardless of nation. Not only factory workers, but bank employees, clerical staffers, and managerial types have been proven, again and again, to be positively affected by music. They work more efficiently and are happier while experiencing the intimate impact of music than when they are deprived. Bars and restaurants, especially in cities, regularly drench their customers in Musak. The impact is gentled; so the listener is never more than half-aware that his emotions are being stroked in this way.

The restaurateur does not wish his customers to hear and therefore listen attentively to music, as such. He wishes them to eat and drink, to consume for their satisfaction and his profit. The human abhorrence of silence is nearly as great as the distress people experience from too much noise or music played so loudly that it becomes noiselike. An individual will enter an empty bar where soft music is playing and remain. He will enter, but soon leave, if no "canned" background music suggests that he is not so much alone, but rather only a bit early. Here the concept of vibration use is continuous, subconscious support rather than stimulation systematized to encourage the responder to remain where he is, within a minienvironment that comforts him and encourages him to consume. These vibrations are more subtle than the Nazi marches, but certainly just as affective and effective as exploitive techniques.

## Speech

Here we shall consider those vocal vibrations that affect human body weather, that is, the intimate impacts of speech on physical health and those psychological states clearly in association.

### Animal Communication

Within this frame, we can order vocal vibrations into four ascending categories: animal, communal, emotional, and intellectual. Those vocalized utterances, usually monosyllabic, that are so similar to the grunts, chirps, and cries of other species, serve the same purposes in man. Animal sounds are physical responses to sensed information about the environment: food or lack of it; comforting shelter; the presence or absence of enemies, associates or peers, mate and offspring; physical discomfort or distress, and the simple powerful emotions of hunger, anger, fear, or lust.

### Chants

Communal vocalized vibrations serve to energize and organize groups for set, short-range activities. The chant, or some longer variation of it, stimulates and sustains collective or cooperative work, itself a physical response to some environmental problem or challenge. Often, these vocalizations are uttered by a single voice, as leader, with a unison response. Presumed to be an early form of speech only slightly more sophisticated than animal utterance, many examples exist today and are found in military, athletic, and religious activities. The noise of machinery has largely replaced communal calls and choruses in the processes of manual labor. While "cheer-leading" as such may be overrated as an energizing signal, the pitch, tempo, cadence, and volume vocalized by the participants rather than the on-lookers is known to make much human activity better coordinated and more rapid and forceful, hence a more efficient conversion of food-fuels into measurable work. The cadenced quality of chanted responses to a leader's cry synchronizes effort with brief periods of rest; the rapid burning of stored glucose is spaced, permitting an increased rate of respiration to bring blood to muscle tissues, minimizing cardiac strain. These sounds enable the strengths of the participants to be shared for purposeful endeavor. They constitute a healthful method of accomplishing tasks in warm climates where the difficulty of heat loss due to high humidity endangers the laboring individual.

## Snarl and Purr Words

Can a human be "scared to death"? Perhaps anecdotal evidence of such exists in some sort of random distribution through the cultures of man. Certainly the power of exorcisms or spoken curses can and does cause debility and death in those who believe that speech itself has supernatural power. More common, everywhere in the modern world, is the observable physical and emotional response to words as commands and to what S. I. Hayakawa has called "snarl and purr words." The polygraph, or lie detector, measures a number of physical responses to speech. The suspect or volunteer is asked questions, and pulse, respiration, blood pressure, and sweating are monitored by electrodes fastened to the body around the chest and arms. Any cry of warning triggers abrupt active response, through the senses to the neuroendocrine system. Fear, as we know, accelerates heartbeat. Often the interval of danger is very brief and the survivor is left with considerable amounts of excess energy and elevated norepinephrine level which prolong a state of physical restlessness accompanied by nervous excitement for as long as an hour after the endangering incident. Anger, the sum of physical and emotional responses to insult or unjust accusation, is exhibited by well-known symptoms: facial flush, engorgement of major muscles with oxygen-rich blood, clenched fists, and rigidity of the jaw and throat musculature to the degree that speech is impaired. Since this condition typically endures longer than fear-responses and the heart must labor to sustain the condition of combativeness, cardiac reserve may be exhausted and insufficiency may cause heart attack. Stroke is another endangering effect associated with argument, anger, and rage. Since joy or surprising pleasure is often triggered by hearing the announcement of our name, this emotion, too, has an impact nearly as powerful as anger, but like anger, often sustained. Heart attack and stroke have turned a great many celebrations and awards festivities into tragic affairs. As conditioners of our own environments, the vocal vibrations of emotion-laden speech have impacts that can literally kill. Normally, the spoken word, either snarled or purred, while a violent affector, does not create life-endangering stress and strain.

## The Communication of Ideas

Speech names, categorizes and abstracts firsthand or vicarious individual or group experiences. Without the utterance, either voiced or muted within, humans cannot and do not think. Speech as an abstractor affects us in different ways. Unlike the animal, communal, or emotional vibration, sound as sense affects us indirectly and over long spans of time. Clearly, this use of man's vocal apparatus is permanently enmeshed within educational processes, both secular and spiritual. Intangibles like "justice," "faith," and "honor" will not affect our physical beings until we have learned what these sounds mean. This sort of vocalized thought reaches back into the individual, group, or national past, skips up to the present time, and rushes into the future—estimating, evaluating, anticipating. Intellectual voices enable us to identify or place ourselves in relation to a group and to time itself. No instruments of measurement have been devised to compile data of an intimate sort resulting from the impacts of voiced thought or sound as idea. Instead, we have what we call history, an *ex post facto* analysis, usually of a cause-effect sort, sometimes biographic in emphasis. These vibrations are enormously powerful and affect whole continents for generations. The vocal cords of man do not vibrate merely to serve his own needs and it is simplistic and dangerous to dismiss political utterance as "a lot of hot air." If humans consider themselves to be an endangered species, who is the enemy?

These considerations of vibrations have moved from noise, scientifically measurable by decibels, to the use and abuse man makes of intermittent, synchronized sequences of controlled pitch. In his own vocalizations, man makes those vibrations that intimately affect himself and others, as their speech affects his physical and mental well-being. Have we moved too far from our central theme of body weather? Not at all.

Simply as vibrations transmitted by air, earth, or water, those indiscriminate, unsynchronized sounds which we call "noise," those intermittent, synchronized, sequenced, harmonized, and controlled sounds we label "music," and the cadenced, standardized, emotive, and information-bearing sounds of our own speech affect every individual, each day of his life. These categories are involved in human work, recreation, love- and war-making, birth and death. Before the trauma of birth, we respond to the steady pulse of our mother's heartbeat transmitted to the unborn brain by the fluids of the womb. We are conceived in the rhythms of the lives of others and die out of those rhythms. The earth we stand on tremors inaudibly. Our planet vibrates on its axis. In a world where whales sing and the percussive touch of a stick on a stretched hide can double the rate of human heartbeat, men and women love and nations perish from the shock of energies unleashed by the quivering of the air we draw in as breath and release as a cry of triumph or despair, how can we deny these vibrations from within and from without as affectors and stressors of our bodies, minds, and souls?

## IRRADIATIONS

As sound of some type is being transmitted constantly on our planet, with man participating as both broadcaster and receiver, so rays of various types and strengths are emitted from a number of sources, both within and beyond our modest solar system. Again, humans broadcast and receive. Individually, we are more likely to be bombarded or penetrated by irradiations than we are to be directly involved in the process of giving off rays more powerful than those that create the electromagnetic field enclosing our bodies. Although we are affected by waves, as well as vibrations, it was not until a bit more than a century ago that we had a name for this condition that affects each of our lives.

### The Electromagnetic Spectrum

The theory of physics was drastically altered and expanded by James Clerk Maxwell's publication of a set of laws describing electric and magnetic phenomena. Central to Maxwell's proof was his demonstration that disturbed conditions at one place could be carried to another place, through space, without a visible transmitter. No matter what the disturbance was, information about it was transmitted elsewhere at the speed of light. Maxwell called the carriers of information "electromagnetic waves," and later research workers have discovered and described their spectrum, which is comparable to the spectrum of natural sunlight. The electromagnetic spectrum not only includes the light rays, but alpha, beta, gamma, and X rays, radio and television waves, and some puzzling emanations from outer space. The length of these waves varies enormously; some are so short that a billion together are no wider than a fingernail, while others are so long they exceed the diameter of the earth by more than twenty times, giving them a wavelength of 186,000 miles. All these are broadcast constantly, although reception is not always equal, either from place to place or at a single site on different days or at different hours. At night, for instance, our earth receives signals that last eight seconds, while the wave cycles of common signals received during the day must be measured in the thousands or tens of thousands per second. Human beings are most evidently responsive to invisible and visible waves of light, located about in the middle of the electromagnetic spectrum, but even though these immensely long waves have very low strengths of field, some forms of life are presumed to be sensitive to them (Watson, 36–37).

Naturally existing radioactive substances undergo nuclear changes that emit three kinds of radiation: alpha waves that are unable to pass through a sheet of common paper, beta waves able to penetrate thin aluminum foil, and energetic gamma rays flashed at the speed of light and capable of passing through moderate thicknesses of lead.

### Natural and Artificial Radiation

Exposure to all sources of radiation is measured in *radiation absorbed dose*, or "rad." In most parts of the world, exposure to radiation from all sources—including the minute emissions from soil, rocks, and various forms of life—has been estimated to average only 100 millirads per year. The individual is likely to be impacted by about three rads in a generation, or probably no more than eight rads in his lifetime.

Since the late 1890s, when the radioactivity of some chemical elements was studied, described, and put to work by scientists, humans in modern technological states have been exposed to very sharp increases in artificial radiation. X rays are a major and preferred diagnostic tool for physicians and dentists. Nuclear changes and radioactivity for most conjure up visions of the atomic bomb and the results of the two blasts unleashed on Japanese civilians during World War II. No less appalling impacts from "fallout" due to testing of nuclear devices in the atmosphere have been photographed and distributed. There are other sources: malfunctioning nuclear reactors, glow-in-the-dark clock and watch dials, microwave ovens, and, of course, the home television set.

Radiation from all natural sources has not increased, so far as can be known. Artificial radiation is a health-affecting factor of our modern environment. Some stars in our universe send out powerful surges of radiation corresponding to the violent changes taking place within them. A lethal dose of cosmic energy for most animals would be about 1,000 roentgen. This has in fact occurred at least three times since life has been on earth. Once, our planet was bombarded briefly by a dose of 2,000 roentgen. The explosions of superstars have irradiated the earth at least a dozen times with enough force to kill most forms of life. Yet, here we all are, as if none of this had happened ( Watson, 36).

### Harmful Radiation

The closer the individual is to a radiation source, the stronger the effect. Radiation loses strength as it passes through human body tissues. The exposure dose on the skin will be higher than the impact of rays on the cells of the pancreas or any other internal organ. What does radiation do? Energy particles strike against and smash the molecules of the cells of the human body. The cells are damaged, but may not be destroyed. Damaged cells either rebuild themselves or are replaced.

Sometimes, for reasons not yet understood, this rebuilding of damaged cells becomes uncontrolled. Regrowth starts, reaches an optimum, and then does not slow down or stop. The cells continue to grow by mitosis at their own best rate. The result is what humans call "cancer."

Radiation can damage the human body in other ways, gradually and invisibly. The effects may not be revealed for decades or more and, by then, may be incorrectly attributed to some more recent cause. If a group of normally healthy humans—say fifty men and fifty women of the same approximate ages—were impacted by a dose of 400 rads that affected the entire body of each, about half the group, or 50 persons, would die in a few months. In a few moments, they had been submitted to more than 100 times the natural exposure of thirty years. This is a tremendous assault on human body cells. The symptoms are anemia, blood poisoning, and internal hemorrhaging. Cells so damaged cannot be repaired or replaced.

A 400-rad dosage administered to an individual over a full thirty years would not cause such a prompt and violent reaction. The likelihood of cancer would increase, though.

Not all human body cells respond to the impact of radiation particles to the same degree. A 400-rad dose distributed over thirty years might prove fatal if the soft, delicate internal organs were directly assaulted. The bombardment of radioactive particles is slowed and weakened by the tougher muscles of the abdomen, however. Some damage results to some cells from any exposure to X-ray irradiation.

A local exposure of thirty rads, ten times the normal exposure of a generation, cannot be felt by the individual at all. Perhaps a week later, the individual, enfeebled by the destruction of blood cells, would be diagnosed as a victim of "radiation sickness."

It has been accepted as a sort of general rule that humans exposed to a dose of twenty rads or less will feel nothing, either at the time of exposure or later. The impact of irradiations is, typically, indirect.

Human body cells can be damaged by radiation so slight that it is measured in thousandths of a rad. This apparently tiny dose can produce significant health changes for the worse: increased tendency to cancer, genetic defects, congenital defects, and premature death.

### Radiation and Birth Defects

The sex cells of men and women contain the code which will determine the characteristics of the children born of union. If a sex cell has been damaged by radiation, the child may be born malformed or with a proclivity toward some disease. These defects may be latent, not visible in the child, but passed on to later generations. Congenital defects can be caused by radiation impact destroying the cells of the unborn child in the mother's womb. Most of the known facts about the effects of radiation impact on human sex cells and unborn infants derive from those Japanese who survived nuclear attack or experienced fallout from atmospheric tests of atomic weapons.

Millirad dosage becomes dangerous, on the global scale, only when some very large group is exposed over a period of time. Human sensitivity to radiation dosage appears to vary as much as does response to vibration. The humans judged to be most vulnerable are persons already sick, the elderly, small children, and the unborn, in that order. When large groups of young adults are exposed to sustained radiation, in millirad dosage, the chances of genetic damage are increased and the likelihood of malformed or vulnerable offspring is also increased.

What is a safe limit for the human individual? About 500 millirads per year. More sensitive individuals are unable to tolerate exposure above 170 millirads, total, annually. These levels are, of course, considerably above that experienced by people from natural environmental irradiation. Persons living within the artificial environments typical of Western technological states are more likely to be exposed to higher, health-impacting levels of millirad exposure. As the years pass, more and more individuals will join the group now living where high millirad exposure from artificial sources is a common, intimate affector of human body weather.

## Health Hazards of X Rays

No one knows when X-ray dosage becomes too much. This invaluable diagnostic tool can actually cause cancer. X rays were regularly used to shrink enlarged thymus glands in infants, until it was discovered that these children later tended to display a high incidence of leukemia and cancer of the thymus. Radiologists, who work daily with X-ray equipment, have a noticeably higher incidence of leukemia than the general public, and higher than any other group of doctors, too. The danger of irradiation, from any source—excessive natural sunlight, radium injections to remedy arthritis of the spine, cobalt bombardment, X rays, television sets, and microovens—comes from the process of *ionization*. Some minimum amount of many kinds of radiation breaks up the molecules of bones, organs, tissues, and cells. No one can say with certainty, "This amount of exposure offers no risk whatever." The effect of impacts is cumulative. While only the seriously ill are involved in regular radiation therapy, the normally healthy sit for months or years of their total life spans exposed to weaker emissions of X rays from home television sets.

Too few people realize that when they watch TV programs, they may be exposing themselves to dangerous levels of radiation from X rays. Most viewers do not think of television sets as low-voltage X-ray machines, which is what they are. The fact is that "Any electronic tube will emit X rays when the voltage applied to it exceeds about 5 kilovolts. Television tubes operate at anywhere from 8 to 25 kilovolts or higher." (Griffiths, 7.)

The National Council of Radiation Protection, an advisory group of scientists (not an agency of the federal government), recommended radiation standards to the government and to television manufacturers in 1960. The maximum permissible rate of X-ray emission from a television set was established at 0.5 millirad per hour, measured at a distance of five centimeters from the surface of the viewing tube. Since X rays weaken in effect (without losing speed) according to the distance from the source, this level was felt to be entirely harmless, especially in view of the fact that most viewers sat about ten feet away, a safe distance. What the Council failed to take into account, however, was that certain age groups typically sit a lot closer to the TV set than a distance of ten feet.

Children, especially, tend to sit too close to television sets, in order to hear broadcast sound lowered to tolerable levels by parents. Public Health Service information, released by the Bureau of Radiological Health in 1971, considered five feet to be the average distance children sit from a television set, just one-half what the NCRP considers safe. Elderly persons who suffer from mild loss of visual acuity or who are hard of hearing tend to sit closer than ten feet away, too. Infants and toddlers crawl around or under home sets and may remain for hours at a distance of less than five feet, when the set is employed as an electronic baby-sitter.

Unfortunately, not only do many children sit closer to television sets than is good for them, they also spend an inordinate amount of their time watching television. In some cultures, children between the ages of two and five watch television for nearly two-thirds of their waking hours. It is also likely that people who grew up during the 1950s, when television sets first became available on a mass scale, spent as much time watching TV programs as they did at work.

As we have seen, the radiation standard suggested by the NCRP for television sets failed to protect the public adequately, but matters were made worse by the number of defective sets flooding the market. In 1964, Japanese researchers monitoring the booming electronics industry that exported so heavily to America reported X-ray emissions over 0.5 millirad per hour in a significant percentage of those television sets using a common form of shunt tube. In 1966, tests at an American assembly plant indicated X-ray leakage impacting workers as they checked new color sets coming off the assembly line. In both instances, the initial concern of researchers, government agencies, and manufacturers was directed toward workers assembling television sets, not purchasers watching sets of the same models tested (Griffiths, 9).

Since the NCRP was not an agency of government, its recommendations did not, and have not, become law. As we have seen, even these minimum standards of safety are measured from the front, the viewer's side of the cathode tube. Actually, this is the area of lowest emission from a defective or dangerous set. X rays from the sides or bottoms of color sets are often ten, hundreds, or thousands of times more powerful than those from the face pointing at the viewer.

What has been done about the thousands of television sets emitting dangerous levels of radiation in American homes? Many of them have been recalled. The *New York Times* of January 11, 1975 carried the following item:

## Wind, Noise, and Irradiation

The Food and Drug Administration has ordered more than 300,000 color television sets manufactured by the Matsushita Electric Corporation of America repaired to correct possibly dangerous radiation levels.

The recall of the sets marketed under the brands Panasonic, J. C. Penney, Pencrest and Bradford is the largest one for television sets in history FDA officials said last night.

Despite such efforts, however, it is a safe bet that many of the television sets found in homes across the land constitute health hazards.

Adverse health effects have been noted among people who watch TV for long periods of time. In 1964 two Air Force physicians presented a report on thirty children, all of whom had been watching television three to six hours a day on weekdays and six to ten hours on Saturdays and Sundays, at a meeting of the American Academy of Pediatrics in New York City. All the children suffered from nervousness, continuous fatigue, headaches, loss of sleep, and vomiting. No explanation for these symptoms could be found after all the customary tests for infectious and childhood diseases had been performed. The upshot was that "the doctors prescribed a total abstinence from TV. In twelve cases the parents enforced the rule and their children's symptoms vanished in two or three weeks." (Ott, 118.)

Radiation does not constitute the only health hazard emanating from TV sets. There are also the programs themselves. Some evidence suggests that the visual and auditory impact of TV programs has undesirable physiological effects. The test recounted below (Carruthers, 82–84) was not intended to be conclusive, but rather exploratory. Since electrocardiogram apparatus measures the heartbeat rate at rest and in response to various stimuli, the ECG records might be considered typical of casual television viewing.

Ten pairs of healthy men and women watched a prerecorded television programme, two couples at a time . . . ECG electrodes were attached and linked . . . outside the viewing room by extended leads. The ECG of each subject in turn could be recorded by rotating the selection switch. . . . the ECG recordings showed significant decrease in minimum heart rate and increase of maximum heart rate, resulting in almost trebling of the gap between the two during the humour, violence and suspense sections of the television programme.

In the environment that we have created for ourselves, it is not possible, really, and most likely not desirable to ban television watching. The millions of sets already in existence and regular operation make testing and recall a practical impossibility. While sociologists and psychologists debate the "information-glut" that tends to devalue any fact, no matter how important, simply because it is but one among so many and deplore the brutalizing effects of televised violence and explicit sex acts, most citizens of any nation transmitting television will not neglect to avail themselves of this "free" source of entertainment and information. Even as the quality of dramatic and comedy programing declines to the nadir of simple-minded tastelessness and repetition, humans tend to accept with a shrug comedian Fred Allen's rueful truth: "If you turn on the faucet and let the water run day and night, you can't complain if the well runs dry."

# 6

# Building Better
# Body Weather

Let me speak to you regarding the things of which you must be
most aware. To get angry and shout at times pleases me, for this
will keep up your natural heat; but what displeases me is your
being grieved and taking all matters to heart. For it is this, as the
whole of physic teaches, which destroys our body more than any
other cause.

> —*Lorenzo Sassoli*

In this chapter, the reader will find a list of recommendations for building better body weather.
No recommendation is, of course, a cure, and it should not be considered as such. In the seventh decade of this century, there is no
shortage of information intended to promote human physical and
mental well-being. The individual reader may wish to investigate
a particular area or to pursue a special interest. A local or regional
library should make this possible at very low cost. At least one book
club and nationally distributed magazine can provide health information with emphasis on prevention, one ounce of which is traditionally worth a pound of cure.

The pages that follow do not assume that the reader has unlimited supplies of time or money. Building better body weather does not require a surplus of either leisure hours or ready cash. Amelioration of your environment may well be limited by the necessities of earning a living. Further, while some environmental factors are obviously under the control of the reader, others are not. Contemporary technology has not only altered life conditions, but the ways and means that must be sought to temper, offset, or remove the negative impacts of environmental influences. Crank attitudes are often fueled by deep fears and frustrations, perhaps invalid readings of experience or too-hasty conclusions drawn from scattered evidence. Fads and fashions in health do not tend to endure long, either for a group or the individual. Often enough, the proponents of a radical alteration of a condition concern themselves more with the style than the substance and cite short-range and dramatic improvements. What we have been concerned with in these pages is the interaction between the human body and the environments that contain it, i.e., long-range effects brought about by the body's response to sustained or seasonal conditions. Change, as such, has not been examined as a cosmetic or as a cure-all, but rather as a natural and typically beneficial stimulus to human health. Finally, we have examined a number of things which affect body weather and have shown that the extremes of any condition are often harmful. The human habit of trying to avoid the ill effects of one condition by total abstinence or absolute denial is of doubtful value in many cases.

## THE GOLDEN MEAN

Since the time of the ancient Greeks, physicians to the body and the mind have urged moderation in all things. Excess and extremes are to be avoided. It appears to be a general truth that what humans call progress has been accomplished at considerable and, in some cases, frightening damage to the planet that supports all life in precarious balance. It is true, also, that our human desire for convenience and comfort has been met with mechanical and electronic devices which have so altered how and where we live that some new "unnatural" health-affecting conditions now exist that were unknown even a generation ago. It is foolish to believe that we can undo all the damage we have inflicted on ourselves and the ecosystems that contain us, while maintaining or increasing the levels of convenience and comfort to which we have grown habituated. As

*150*

we can be said to have unwittingly inflicted upon ourselves conditions which triggered the general adaptation syndrome, it is only reasonable to believe that similar responses would be caused if we reversed the processes of progress. We cannot and will not return to our own past styles and solutions; there is no evidence to indicate that any such attempt would benefit anybody.

What seems sensible then, is for each individual to seek moderate means to build better body weather without recourse to expensive gadgets, radical changes in life-style, or total reorganization of the modes of work and recreation. What is suggested is manipulations from a moderate base, making the best uses of what is available. The best monitor and controller of physical and mental health is the self, not some external authority or prescription. Better body weather is obtainable by what you can do with yourself for yourself. It may mean retraining to give up some habits adjudged to be harmful, but accept as a truth that humans do not easily abandon any practice, even for good cause. What appears to be more effective is to consider learning some new habits likely to do you some real good if maintained for years, even decades. The weather, as we all know, is sufficiently changeable that if we don't care for it, all we have to do is wait for it to alter. Climate, as we have seen, is the sum of many conditions affecting life over long spans of time—a range of changes, really. Accept this, and you may find that you are more comfortably attuned, able to accept the changes in your own body weather within the climate of your lifetime.

## YOUR DIET AND YOUR HEALTH

One significant step you may want to take is the adoption of a nutrition plan suitable for your needs, body-type, age, sex, and general health history. In these pages, we have considered at length the effects and impacts of forces outside the body. Clearly, what we call the diet is a major affector of human physical and mental well-being. What is inside the body and put there by you is now and will be a major factor of your body weather. We do not deal with this matter fully here because of the problem of length, not indifference. Diet and nutrition make up a large subject area that would require another book to treat several points of view fairly. Human diet is not only critical, but controversial.

Decide to take better care of your body by learning more about your physical apparatus. It may have been many years since you took a science course in school, and it is quite likely that you are under- or misinformed about the facts of nutrition. Accept as a sad truth that the average family doctor is not likely to be much better informed than you are. Investigate and inform yourself about nutrition facts, taking care to read several books, not just one at random or on the recommendation of a friend. As in all processes of learning, small but regular exposure to contemporary thinking is likely to produce confident awareness, while a "crash course" may leave you muddled.

Be certain of your words. "Diet" is a sort of climate, the sum of factors over a long period of time. Physicians and researchers study and write of diet in the national sense, often measuring impacts over decades or generations. In popularized usage, this word really means a regimen designed to encourage weight-loss in a relatively brief time span. Forget about diet in the popular sense. No individual should undertake a regimen of weight-loss without the advice and consent of a physician. Any number of ten-day or thirty-day programs are essentially cosmetic, designed to make the individual *look* better (that is, slimmer). Your interest should be in controlling food-fuel intake to make you *feel* better. Some regimens require drinking a lot of water or taking in very little liquid. Some contemporary regimens are innovative, unproven, and of dubious value, even dangerous. The American Medical Association has publicly condemned those regimens urging people to curtail intake of carbohydrates so sharply as to effectively eliminate this category of food. Read, reflect, become self-informed, but do not undertake a major alteration in the kinds of food that you eat. Certainly consult a doctor before attempting to lose weight. You may not need to, and the attempt to shed twenty pounds might be harmful.

### Harmful Additives

There is little disagreement concerning the kinds of chemical additives with which modern man douses his food both during the manufacturing processes and at the table. A number of compounds are introduced in the processing of foods to improve color or to prolong shelf-life. These additives benefit the seller, not the consumer. The two common table additives, sugar and salt, so liberally sprinkled over almost everything, are often unnecessary and quite unnatural; that is, the use of these substances has been learned from the culture, not dictated by the requirements of the human body or mind.

In 1968, figures released by the United States government

indicated that each American, regardless of age or condition of health, consumed ninety-eight pounds of sugar in the preceding year. Since then, national consumption has risen. Sugar use is very high in all technologically advanced nations. Just over ten years ago, Professor John Yudkin published two articles in the prestigious medical journal, *The Lancet*, in which he questioned the significance of the correlation of dietary fats with high incidence of heart disease, suspecting that this was an association rather than a cause-effect link. Professor Yudkin argued that correlations could be made between increased incidence of a number of diseases and increased consumption of refined sugar. Of all foods, refined sugar has shown the most rapid rise in rate of consumption in wealthy countries. Yudkin cited reports issued by the United Nations, elaborate investigations of the diet of nations and subgroups. Yudkin's views were not warmly received by makers of ice cream, pastries, and precooked foods, or by medical specialists who favor the cholesterol theory of heart disease. Nevertheless, his conclusions and observations have been very widely reprinted, discussed, and cited. A good deal of evidence supports his view. It is quite likely that the average Canadian or American should reduce sugar consumption, eliminating the refined product at the table and substituting honey or molasses out in the kitchen. Any person reading extensively in health books and journals is likely to come across Yudkin's name. His studies of patients suffering from arterial diseases revealed that those sufferers were in the habit of consuming, on the average, twice as much refined sugar daily as the members of a disease-free control group. Overdosage of sugar, as a "climate," is harmful to the human heart ( Rodale, *Diet*, 69–81).

Salt, the other common additive, is believed by most persons to be good for the system, especially on a hot, muggy day. The folk belief persists that heavy labor or very active recreation demands immediate replacement of salt sweated from the system. Self-administration of two or more salt tablets is unwise, however, since it overloads the system with sodium chloride and speeds the loss of potassium from the body. Potassium depletion can lead to heat prostration. More than fifteen years ago, test results published in *Current Therapeutic Research* indicated that 87 percent of a small test group reported significant improvement in health when administered potassium. Complaints of headache, fatigue, local pain, sleeplessness, and lowered sexual drive were reduced. While humans do need a small amount of salt, they need potassium, too. About 2.5 grams of salt per day from all sources seems to be about what adult humans need for health. Americans consume a great deal more, as an additive and preservative, then often sprinkle additional amounts on at the table, for daily totals twice, three times or more above need (Rodale, *Diet*, 151).

Excessively high salt intake, which has a cumulative effect over the years, is associated with kidney failure, enlarged heart, and hypertension in humans. Laboratory animals reveal disastrous results in a matter of months. The relationship between human salt intake and blood pressure increase appears to be proportionate. Common table salt causes all human tissues to retain water inside the cells. This water causes weight-gain. Obesity itself is a danger to the heart, as we have seen. Sodium-reduced or restricted regimens are common, and the list of prohibited foods is a formidable one, since it contains so many of the convenience preparations and snacks that well-to-do Westerners have learned to substitute for natural fruits, nuts, and vegetables.

### Minerals and Fibers

One sure result of a self-generated program of reading in the area of health, diet, and nutrition will be a new supply of helpful information on human mineral requirements. You may be pleased to learn that you are already providing your physical apparatus with its overall requirements, year round. You are likely to discover that some foods are worthy of more regular appearances on your plate since they contain significant amounts of certain minerals very likely to provide better body weather in some surprising ways. Zinc, for instance, as well as potassium. Some recent work in the field of biochemistry has been published indicating likely preventive benefits from mineral-rich foods, with secondary benefits if consumed in the raw state.

Already, books and magazine articles have publicized the health gains that can be obtained, at very low cost and little inconvenience, from a self-controlled intake of foods containing natural fibers. This has made the manufacturers of certain whole wheat, bran, and granola-type cereals very happy. Eating such foods can make you more healthy, but not necessarily slimmer. Regimens designed to encourage weight loss are difficult to sustain. A more natural diet is easy to get on and stay on. The foods themselves taste good, and as you reduce your daily intake of additives, especially refined sugar and salt, the natural flavors become especially pleasurable. In the long run, you are certain that your diet is creating the best conditions inside your body for better body weather. Your diet has become a "climate" for good health. High-fiber foods do, in fact, offer a measure of protection from serious diseases, illnesses especially prevalent in advanced, technological nations.

It is a fact worth noting that a good deal of this "new" information about healthful minerals and natural fibers has been in the hands of the readers of the major health and nutrition magazine for well over a decade. The magazine is *Prevention*. Some physicians fuss about the "bias" of *Prevention*'s editorial policy, because the magazine is resolutely opposed to the easy, too casual habit of prescribing drugs as a cure, while both physicians and patients ignore the healthful benefits of good nutrition and regular, moderate exercise. The magazine investigates and reports on a wide range of health information. Its "bias," in the face of our drug-conscious society's relentless promotion of chemical compounds, is a sane attempt to create a balance between excesses and extremes, hence a balance that enables readers to obtain and sustain good body weather.

## EXERCISE, FITNESS, AND BODY WEATHER

To the best of your opportunities and within the limits set by the climate, weather, and conditions where you live, a self-controlled program of *regular, moderate* exercise will create and maintain a degree of physical fitness that is likely to offset the minor lapses from a healthful diet. You may recall Coronaro's advice for longevity: temperance and exercise. He was not advocating total abstinence and athletic training, but self-governed moderation. About the same time—that is, over 300 years ago—the Englishman John Dryden wrote:

> Better to hunt in fields for health unbought
> Than fee the doctor for nauseous draught,
> The wise, for cure, on exercise depend;
> God never made his work for man to mend.

You can hunt your fields for health, too, certain that a moderate, regular program of outdoor exercise promotes body weather in three ways: improving muscle tone, adapting the body to seasonal change, and exposing the body to full-spectrum natural sunlight to offset possible malillumination effects caused by excessive exposure to artificial light sources. No doctor, no publication, no true friend will urge violent exercise on weekends, followed by five days of dietary excess and physical sloth. A program for prevention of disease should not be a purge-and-splurge cycle or one likely to cause breakdown or accidents, including coronary accidents as well as strains and sprains. The wonders of drugs have overshadowed the benign and inexpensive health benefits that can be found through exercise. Cardiac rehabilitation programs now encourage participants to retrain damaged hearts through exercise, under supervision and with due caution.

Consider the fact that most forms of regular and inexpensive exercise do what helps, but not what harms. A low-sugar, low-salt, high-fiber diet plus moderate exercise builds health and strength without strain. Assaulting the human bowels with a high-starch and sugar-drenched diet and making them additionally costive by lack of activity make the everyday need for evacuation of human wastes a heart-straining period of work. Human blood pressure soars when the body strains to effect bowel movement, often higher than most forms of exercise (Carruthers, 107).

Many other high-risk conditions that threaten health and life (high blood fat level, elevated blood pressure, intolerance for sugar, too rapid blood clotting) have been found to decrease in both men and women who take the few moments per day needed to maintain a fitness training program. If you exercise you are certain to feel better, look better, work better, relax more easily, and sleep more soundly. All this without expensive equipment or costly drugs. Such a program will not only aid in curing what ails you, but will substantially reduce your chances of heart attack.

**How to Determine Your Maximum Safe Heartbeat**

Take the number 200 and subtract your age in years. The result will be the top of the range for your heartbeat rate per minute, if you are now in reasonable good health. That is, a sound person fifty years of age should regard 150 beats per minute (200–50) as the maximum level at which his heart should be permitted to beat, while exercising. Isometric exercises, which tend to elevate blood pressure and increase the cardiac work-load, should be avoided. Don't lift weights and don't do pushups. Unless you are a professional football player, collegiate athlete in training or about to join an alpine team, you run the risk of harming yourself and your heart.

Avoid masochistic or maximal efforts at anything. If it hurts, quit and rest. If you feel exhausted during or after, cut back or cut it out, at once. Physical training programs in a gymnasium are seldom run by therapists familiar with the special needs of the physically *unfit*. You do not need a "body-building" program or a "slimnastics" set of exercises in competition with others offered once a week. Below is an evaluation of some popular, easily accessible forms of exercise, from the health-benefit point of view.

### Walking

Walking is mild stimulation and promotes good circulation, respiration, and healthful appetite. Most likely, it does not strengthen the heart muscle so much as it prevents weakness. Walking is excellent for out-of-shape humans, as a rehabilitator after heart attack, and for fitness maintenance. By itself, walking is probably not a preventer of disease, but rather a good conditioner in conjunction with sound diet.

### Jogging

A preferred type of exercise for would-be athletes (or has-beens), jogging is presently a popular, even fashionable type of exercise. However, as a health promoter, jogging has been over-rated. Severe stress is likely, especially for persons overweight. Self-monitored jogging is difficult to maintain as a program, since the individual tends to trot longer distances or to traverse the same distance in less time. Cold-weather jogging raises both blood pressure and fat levels in the human blood. Jogging with others tends to become competitive and increases the flow of adrenaline and norepinephrine to levels normally associated with severe physical labor or powerful emotional reactions.

### Swimming

Better body weather is promoted by noncompetitive swimming. A varied, pleasant social form of exercise, it is subject to better self-control. Essentially isotonic exercise, the tension of muscles remains about the same and some of the work of movement is reduced by the fact that the body is buoyed by water. All the muscles of the body are exercised, a distinct gain over either walking or jogging. For the cosmetically conscious, swimming is slimming. Cold water is a shock to the human system and triggers the mechanisms that release extra fat into the blood to provide needed body heat. The secret here is not to overdo the length of swimming, since body heat loss is about fifteen times greater in water than in still air at the same temperature. Membership in an indoor, heated pool club is a good way to swim, year-round, without ruinous expense. YMCA/ YWCA or YMHA/YWHA facilities exist in most cities and costs are modest. Body weather swimming is not racing, and the basic rule of 200 minus your age in years must set the top level of heartbeat rate. Discomfort and chill are to be avoided, as is exhaustion.

### Squash and Tennis

These popular racket games have the very great disadvantage of being stop-and-go sports: peaks of violent activity, a lot of muscle, tendon, and joint strain, plus emotional stress from competition. Heartbeat rates swing erratically, making for a health cost that may match the wallet-drain of membership in a club for indoor play. Weekend tennis is hard to "get in shape" for, and late-maturity adults can swat their way through the season and accomplish no gain that might be regarded as health-maintaining.

### Golf

There are so many stories, jokes, anecdotes, and descriptions of this game and the vagaries of playing it, that it seems almost unfair to point out that it is extraordinarily expensive, without being especially health-promoting. It is less stimulating than a steady three-mile walk at a good pace. The exercise of the swing is violent and straining to the human frame, and the degree of coordination required is so precise that golf is a game of excruciating frustration and surprising mood swings. And the "nineteenth hole" is a hazard that may be worse than all the sand traps and deep rough combined.

### Cycling

The bicycle is back, both as a response to the rise in gas prices and as a pollution protest. Not only is the bicycle a valuable system of transportation, but its health benefits are real, despite the accident-risk of highway use. New gear systems like the *derailleur* effectively reduce, if not remove, the steep hills and permit even the novice biker to pedal five miles a day and hop off stimulated, but unstressed and unstrained. A varied and social activity, it can be practiced for a lifetime on three wheels or two. The expense of purchasing a good-quality bike is initial only, with low-cost maintenance. Temperate-zone pedalers may have to put the machine on a storage rack in very cold weather and moderate use in inclement weather, when rain makes pavements slippery. Year-round, it probably costs less than membership in a swimming club. Cycling is a regular isotonic exercise, deservedly popular with humans of all ages and non-polluting. City-dwellers may have traffic and atmospheric conditions that suburbanites do not encounter with such severity, but park trails and bike routes are increasing, even within the "heat-island" microclimates.

If exercise is now your habit, keep it up and look for ways to convert the stressful start-and-stop games to those activities providing moderate stimulation at sustained levels that can be endured on every occasion year after year. If exercise is not your habit, you can build better body weather (not a better body in the Mr. Muscle sense) by taking up some form that is pleasant, personally enjoyable, and easily available where you live and where you choose to vacation. Good exercise should be fun, something that can be shared, with no prizes to win except some new friends, perhaps. As for costs, keep them at common-sense levels, easily affordable on your present income and after retirement. You should not have to buy into exercise or find yourself priced out. Your choice should be pretty much climate-proof, suitable for about 300 days of the year, and something you can and like to do. Maybe, for most persons, walking is the ideal solution and the most natural form of activity at lowest cost. Millions walk for pleasure and health, convinced that it promotes their best body weather.

## SENSIBLE TEMPERATURE CONTROL

You know you can't function at your best in overheated indoor spaces; so control thermostat settings accordingly. Indoor readings of sixty-five degrees Fahrenheit permit comfort without feelings of suffocation or "baking." Humidity needs to be monitored, too. Humans seem to function most efficiently when the humidity is about 40 percent. In northern areas of the temperate zone, the cold exterior air makes humans turn up the heat in early fall and leave it up until late spring or early summer. Humidity control during that many months prevents delicate throat and nasal membranes from drying out. In any cool climate, adding moisture to indoor air does not require expensive equipment. Perhaps your grandmother set a bowl or pan of water on the radiator in every room, refilling them once a week, as slow evaporation took place. This combination of moderate temperature and deliberate moisturizing of the air avoids extreme conditions known to be harmful to human physical health and alert mental well-being.

### Natural Ways to Adjust to Seasonal Weather Change

Precondition yourself for winter cold, beginning in late summer. A regular exercise program, out of doors, will combine a fitness plan and preconditioning at the same time. Instead of avoiding the exterior climate, make use of the natural environment in a natural way. This does not mean reckless exposure to chill or heavy rain. Instead of bundling under layers of wool or artificial fibers, underdress slightly and then allow moderate exercise like walking or riding a bike combine with air temperature to stimulate your combustion rate, bringing body heat up to the level of comfort. If you sweat, then you are wearing too much; if you shiver, you are not wearing enough. Beginning early, when it's still warm enough to go swimming, will enable your physical responses to adjust to the natural environment as the season changes. Perhaps for the first time, you will be using weather to promote your own health, employing seasonal change as an ally, rather than fleeing from the local weather as an enemy.

Use common sense and do not ride a bike or go jogging in severe cold. Wind-chill impacts can become severe stress very quickly, and moderate exercise becomes hard work, kicking up your heartbeat rate and releasing fats into the bloodstream. A brisk walk in hat, jacket, and gloves will stimulate your body without undue and unwanted strain. Let your nose warn you. You should be able to breathe easily, without any sensation of discomfort. If the air seems to "ache," it's too cold. In your everyday walks use two city blocks or a half-mile as your personal stress-test. With that amount of warmup time, you can judge your own experience. If the impacts of air and wind are causing discomfort, go home. Habituation is one thing, suffering is another. The trick is to begin this process before it seems necessary; so do not pick an arbitrary calendar date. Remember that the nature of weather is change and that weather always is in the process of becoming something else. Exposing yourself to environmental stimulus is an ancestral technique and it takes some relearning. You may have some slight adjustments to make in the fall (most persons acclimatizing themselves tend to overdress), but in the late winter you will be an early sensor of the approaching spring. Do not think of acclimatizing as a "toughening" process or you'll start to punish yourself. Moderation and regularity, with adjustments, should be the watch words, both indoors and out. No one will accuse you of being a "fresh air fiend," and rush to take your photo as you break a hole in the ice to go swimming in mid-January. Rather, you will live in a slightly cooler home or apartment with optimum humidity that you manipulate. Outdoor temperatures will be slightly less shocking, and everyday acclimatization will have you still in a sweater or light coat while others shiver beneath heavier wrappings. After all, what does clothing really do? Dress traps and slows body heat loss. English, European, and American polar explorers suffered cruelly, until they adopted the Eskimo garb of loose skin parkas over bare skin, so that released body heat formed a comfortable layer of warm air. Keep this in mind. Too snug winter dress defeats its own purpose. Too tight sweaters, blouses, or jackets transmit body heat, rather than trapping a layer of body-warmed air, Eskimo style.

In the spring and summer, reverse the process, acclimatizing to warmer conditions by daily exposure but always within your best range of comfort. Avoid the stresses of severe heat and humidity when out of doors. Underdress slightly and move around. Sweating is an emergency sign that you should heed. Slow down, seek the shelter of shade, and look for a breeze.

## Comfortable Cooling

Better body weather has become yours when you are not conscious of feeling either chilled or overheated. As a general rule, when you are conscious of your own physical envelope in response to conditions around you, it is a form of discomfort likely to impair your efficiency to some extent. You should be acclimated so that you are really unaware of your body in relationship to the immediate environment. Then, fine coordination of body muscles and improved concentration of the mind are much more possible. You will want to avoid, then, the midsummer chills of excessive and unmodulated air conditioning, at work and at home. The humidity can slide up to about 75 percent, if the air temperature in your office is, say, eighty degrees Fahrenheit. Conversely, if you set your home unit for seventy degrees and permit humidity to match it, you'll have the sensation of living inside a fog bank or a low cloud formation. These conditions of real discomfort are more common in huge office complexes, where interior weather is crudely manipulated with a single setting for an entire building or whole floor.

Again, since your aim is a state of comfort and your body is the master sensor, ignore the calendar, but this time keep an eye on the thermometer registering the outdoor temperature. Do not be a victim of the "set-and-forget" school of climate control. Adjust temperature for comfort about ten degrees Fahrenheit below external conditions. An artificial "uniseason" is unnatural and stressing. Better body weather is a self-controlled acclimatization to seasonal changes. At all times seek comfort for optimum efficiency, but never June in January or vice versa.

## HOW TO ADJUST TO CHANGES IN AIR PRESSURE

The one aspect of the weather not subject to your personal control is atmospheric pressure changes. Here the motto is an old one: "If you can't lick 'em, join 'em." Your body is as sensitive to the rise and fall of atmospheric pressures as it is to temperature and humidity, but you cannot sense your own responses in such immediate and physical ways. The feelings you will have manifest themselves from the inside out, so to speak. A falling barometer is likely to be accompanied by mildly depressed moods and mental states. Nothing serious, just the "blahs." Do not kick up the air conditioner and attempt to "snap out of it" by chilling yourself. Increased heat in the winter won't do you any good either. Ride with the change. The body is supposed to respond; attempts to triumph over the natural environment are foolish. Two cups of coffee are likely to make you feel jittery without making you feel better. Psychological states with physical responses associated with atmospheric pressure are natural and necessary. If your mind shuts down slightly, let it. Benefit from your own body weather warnings. If problems arise, side-step those not so urgent, but set a time to resolve the issues: "First thing tomorrow." Humans tend to lose problem-solving efficiency when the barometer falls. Why attempt the difficult, when you are not naturally attuned? Trust yourself. A delay in decision-making gives your slowed mentality more time to weigh alternatives.

Listen to weather forecasts, not merely to learn temperature and likelihood of rain. Is the barometer holding steady, on the rise, or falling? If it's on the way down, and you know this early in the morning, rearrange your work so that demanding tasks are undertaken before noon. If you can anticipate weather changes outside yourself, you can and should anticipate the internal changes in your body weather. Psychologically, it's a nice feeling to know that you've controlled the utilization of your skills and timed your efforts to coincide with natural efficiency peaks. You will feel much better about yourself coasting through a dull, depressing afternoon with the demanding work behind you.

Pressure changes cause mood swings. If you anticipate your own, you will be in a better state to tolerate the cranky irritability and inefficiency of others. It is unwise to try to medicate against moods, when the weather is the prime cause of depressed physical and mental states.

## DRUG DANGERS

Better body weather should come from sensitive and sensible acclimatization, temperate and informed diet and exercise. You can't buy good body weather in a bottle. Be very cautious about allowing your body and mind to learn habits that harm more than they help. For every low there is a corresponding high, in the natural environment, that is, not through drug use. You can make yourself feel worse by attempting to dose your way out of depression with another cup of coffee, just one more pill, or an extra drink. Even a sudden surrender to refined sugar may leave you feeling worse than before.

Be aware, too, that factors like heat, humidity, and atmospheric pressure have sufficiently strong impacts as to alter responses to medications your physician may have prescribed. There is reason to believe that basic metabolic processes involving vitamin absorption and utilization are altered by weather changes. You have to expect and to respect the changes that are natural outside and inside your body. Modern man has a tendency to push himself, to believe that overstimulation is good because it seems to use time more productively. Make up your mind whether you want to be rich, once, for a short time or healthy through the course of a long and useful life. While medical records abound concerning breakdown, disability, and premature death resulting from drug abuse, there is a norm, and that is the kind of self-controlled and self-monitored body maintenance that can be effected through a low-sugar, low-sodium, high-fiber diet combined with regular moderate exercise in deliberate acclimated response to the natural environment. There is some evidence that supplementary vitamins and certain minerals help improve the natural efficiency of bodily systems. These are not stimulants or stressors.

**Cigarettes**

Cigarettes are air pollution by the pack. What most people need to do is simply heed the warning from the Surgeon General printed on the side of every package. There is reason to believe that persons over sixty years of age can give up the smoking habit with less fuss and hysteria than younger men and women. Perhaps the awareness of reduced time in the future creates a stronger motivation to live out one's remaining years with uncontaminated lungs. Quitting is harmless to the health, after all, and fear of sudden weight-gain is irrational. If you can exercise the self-control needed to avoid system-poisoning excesses of sugars and starches, success in that area will strengthen determination to kick the cigarette habit.

**Alcohol**

Alcohol continues to be the most abused drug on the continent of North America. The insidious nature of alcohol itself and the unknowable levels of individual tolerance make it a risky compound, although long-sanctioned by our culture as a kind of "natural" cure-all. Dependence very easily becomes addiction, and the user is "hooked" before becoming consciously aware of the fact. No one deliberately becomes an alcoholic, and addiction to this drug is an accident, but one with very powerful aftereffects and side-effects, too. Although some wines are judged to contain limited amounts of natural vitamins, distilled alcohol is simply a chemical with empty calories. Alcohol stimulates the release of neutral fats into the blood, and too much affects the nervous system. For many, alcohol is the preferred tranquilizer, but it is a depressant after a first quick "high." Many physicians are poorly trained in recognizing the disease of alcoholism and will prescribe sedative compounds or tranquilizers that are themselves subject to abuse. Polyaddiction to drug compounds *and* alcohol is a relatively new phenomenon and extremely dangerous.

Alcohol has been used by man to warm up and to cool off for several centuries. To some degree, it does both, insofar as it dilates the blood vessels and eases circulation to the skin, permitting rapid heat-loss. Finally, however, it dulls or depresses self-awareness. The drinker does not feel the cold so severely, although he is likely to freeze to death faster than a sober individual. Cold beer or an icy gin and tonic makes the drinker feel cool and promotes sweating, both temporary states. Generally speaking, the use of alcohol as a manipulator of body weather and mood swings is inefficient, expensive, fattening and, if pleasant for many, potentially dangerous for about one person in ten. As the rain falls on the just and the unjust alike, drug addiction is extremely democratic. You have no way of knowing what your responses to drugs may be, either in the short or the long term. This fact alone should encourage people to consider chemical compounds as medications solely for prescribed use in the case of serious sickness or degenerative disease.

## HOW TO GET YOUR HEALTH FROM OTHER PEOPLE

While it seems true that we contract infectious diseases from other people, depending on our own state as potential host to the microorganisms, we respond more strongly to other humans as conditioners of our environments. We rightly use metaphors such as "infectious laughter" and "voice of doom" to describe our physical and emotional reactions to other people. While most of us are content to make and maintain rather minimal human contacts, "seeing the same old friends," we are enlivened, not just entertained, by fresh contacts. Strangers are naturally stimulating people; they challenge us to communicate, to respond and share. Men and women in normal, natural good health transmit some of their exuberance and confidence to those around them. We can "catch" a cold from an acquaintance, but we can catch enthusiasm, too. Genuine contact with humanity face to face is more enlivening both physically and mentally than second-hand contact. Television, especially, is a surrogate and, for some, a habit. The set serves too many as a kind of drug, and they are addicted to their electronic companion. This condition is very evident among retirees and the elderly, and the symptoms of television addiction are close to those that mark clinical depression: physical inactivity, decreased willingness to communicate with other persons, and a proclivity to skip meals or to abandon health-sustaining diet.

Again we see that the total environment offers a choice: the natural and the artificial, stimulating changes or standardized imitation. Once the artificial assumes a position of dominance over human responses, replacing natural affectors, some measure of self-control over our own body weather is sacrificed. Television personalities are inadequate substitutes for real human beings. The "vibrations" of family, friends, neighbors, and strangers stimulate us in ways no television program can. We can dial ourselves some temporary illusions, but we cannot tune out the impacts of external life conditions, even if we remain too much and too long indoors.

## ULTRAVIOLET THERAPY

A paper submitted to a symposium at the University of Oregon Medical School back in 1965 seems to summarize the antisunlight school of thought:

> It has been suggested that prolonged exposure to sunlight may result in the development of skin cancer in man. . .

Sunburn is an excess, an extreme, and to be avoided. Prolonged sun exposure dries human skin and causes premature aging of tissues, just the reverse of the healthy tanned look many people seek. The heat from too much direct sun can cause prostration.

Dr. Ellinger, author of *Medical Radiation Biology*, submits that the full spectrum of natural sunlight (both visible and invisible rays) is of direct benefit to man. What is more to the point, he was able to measure the benefits using cardiovascular responses as indicators of improved work-output and decreased fatigue (Ott, 93):

> Irradiation of human subjects with . . . doses of ultraviolet resulted in improved work output. In studies on the bicycle ergometer [which measures the amount of work done by a group of muscles under control conditions] it has been shown that the work output could be increased up to 60% . . . due to decreased fatigability and increased efficiency.

Three Russian scientists, reporting to a meeting of the International Committee on Illumination in Washington, D.C. in 1967, supported Ellinger's position with comments of their own (Ott, 94):

> If human skin is *not* exposed to solar radiation . . . for long periods of time, disturbances will occur in the . . . equilibrium of the human system . . . functional disorders of the nervous system and a vitamin D deficiency, a weakening of the body's defenses, and an aggravation of chronic diseases. Sunlight deficiency is observed more particularly in persons . . . working underground or in windowless industrial buildings.
>
> The simplest and at the same time most effective measure for the prevention of this deficiency is the irradiation of human beings by means of ultraviolet lamps. . . . As a rule, the average dosage of ultraviolet does not exceed half of the average dose which produces a just perceptible reddening of the untanned human skin.

*166*

Sunlight therapy for Russian workers is, apparently, very carefully controlled to promote better body weather, not for cosmetic effects.

Millions of Canadians and Americans suffer from the annoying disease of psoriasis. As the condition is believed to be genetic, the most effective countermeasure is a treatment, not a cure. Psoriasis seems to have its own annual cycle, improving during the spring and summer, erupting into disfiguring, itchy patches in the winter. A four-man team combining Harvard Medical School and Massachusetts General Hospital personnel developed an oral dose of methoxsalen, a compound known to the ancient Egyptians. They administered this to patients, then exposed them to long-wave ultraviolet. Lesions have vanished and once-weekly maintenance treatments control further outbreaks. Additional tests in Europe confirm this phototherapy.

## Sun Lamps

Be wary of commercial "sun lamps," and check with the retailer before purchase. Some emit energy peaks of *short*-wave ultraviolet (normally filtered out by the atmosphere). Look for the word "germicidal" on the box or in the how-to-use copy. Short-wave ultraviolet slows the reproduction of some kinds of microorganisms. This sort of lamp is dangerous, since it can cause severe burns and other tissue injuries.

## UVT Bulbs and Tubes

You can obtain ultraviolet-transmitting bulbs and fluorescent tubes manufactured by the Duro-Test Corporation for installation in offices, factories, school rooms, and the home. "Daylight white" fluorescent tubes make reptiles more active, and seem to stimulate laboratory mice. Animal fertility rises, and at least one zookeeper has attributed increases in animal population to UVT lights installed in zoo facilities.

In the winter of 1968–69, the "Hong Kong flu" struck the United States. The Florida Health Department reported 6,000 cases in Sarasota, a major resort and retirement area. Two sections of Sarasota Memorial Hospital were shut down, since more than sixty of the hospital's nurses were ill from the disease. A few miles away, at Obrig Laboratories, not one employee missed a day's work due to the disease. Obrig Laboratories operated inside the first plant in

America designed with both full-spectrum illumination and ultra-violet-transmitting window materials (Ott, 105).

While you might not wish to invest in replacing all your windows with UVT panes, changing indoor illumination by replacing conventional bulbs with Duro-Test products is a step most persons can take to bring full-spectrum sunlight inside their offices and homes. Children, especially, seem to benefit from UVT illumination.

### UVT Glass for Eyeglasses

You may wish to consider John Ott's experiences with phototherapy or disregard what has been called "anecdotal evidence." It will cost you nothing to sit in the shade wearing neither prescriptive glasses nor dark lenses of conventional glass, both of which screen out ultraviolet. Not all opticians carry UVT materials for grinding into prescriptive lenses, and some vigorously promote their inventories of "glare-reducing" dark glasses. A little information passed along might encourage your optician to learn more than he now knows about the apparent health benefits from ultraviolet long waves. Involved with remedying defective vision, he may have forgotten or chosen to ignore that setting conventional glass between the environment and the human eye is quite contrary to nature and that prolonged, everyday use of regular glass must necessarily affect the neuroendocrine system to some degree. Perhaps he, and you, will opt to replace conventional glass in your eyeglasses with UVT glass.

## NOISE POLLUTION

According to new information reported by the National Institute for Occupational Health and Safety, two or three years of daily exposure to vibration or sound at the ninety-decibel level is sufficient to induce deafness to some degree. Impacts of seventy decibels are potentially damaging if exposure is quite prolonged, say ten years in an office where business machines clatter and heavier equipment nearby vibrates as well. The noise level in most major cities in the United States equals or exceeds 70 decibels daily and seldom falls below this level.

The National Research Council in Canada reports that about 35 million Americans live in areas where the *average* noise holds at sixty-five decibels. While this level may not be harmful, it is annoying. Perhaps 90 percent of Americans are assaulted by vibrations above 75 decibels. The World Health Organization estimates that noise costs in dollar terms, too, about $4 billion annually due to accidents, absenteeism, and compensation claims. The impacts of noise and music must be considered as stressors. "Bad vibes" are believed to impair sexual functioning, induce fatigue, cause weight loss, and excite ulcers and high blood pressure. While the evidence is not conclusive, many urban dwellers live complete lifetimes in a microclimate that ceaselessly batters at their senses, impacting their bodies in ways for which the human body and nervous system have not evolved defenses (*New York Times Magazine*, 23 November, 1975, p. 31).

Not all persons can move out of the urban "heat-islands" and others do not choose to do so. Urbanites tend to move up to higher levels in order to escape the assault of noise. This is a self-controlled treatment, but not a cure, and one that is limited, unfortunately, to those affluent enough to pay higher rents. The rural poor are not afflicted with noise pollution, since countryside sound levels rarely peak above 40 decibels. Both urban and rural populations experience malnutrition, and Dr. Samuel Rosen at New York's Mt. Sinai Hospital believes that such conditions may explain why partial deafness may be so common in technological communities or "advanced nations." A great deal of attention has been directed to the diet of African nations and Dr. Rosen is among those who noted Sudanese tribes in good health, nourished by high-fiber foods, low in animal or dairy fats, but adequate in protein, vitamins, and minerals. This group had hearing acuity far above that typical of industrial America (*New York Times Magazine*, 23 November, 1975, p. 70).

### How to Reduce Noise Levels

You may not need to migrate away from excessive noise levels at work and at home. You can check your responses to noise without counting decibels. If your pulse rate increases and you find yourself feeling edgy, aggressive, and irritable, it may be that the noise around you has crept up over 75 decibels. You may have "gotten used to it" intellectually, but your body responds negatively. Inexpensive sound-damping or sound-proofing materials are available at local hardware stores. Thick curtains, wall hangings, and carpeting all absorb large amounts of indoor racket.

If possible without real inconvenience or added cost, exercise by walking or cycling in areas that moderate urban noise. A stroll down a city street may expose you to more noise than you can comfortably tolerate—roaring traffic, the batter of pavement-breakers, and blaring music from a dozen transistor radios. A subway token can take you to another section of the city, but you may not enjoy the ride.

Remember that music is a powerful affector of physical and emotional responses. Too often, it is used as a kind of jamming system or sonic gag to blot out background commotion. It should and can relax you, besides promoting feelings of tranquility and harmony. Many adults believe, incorrectly, that contemporary radio broadcasting is limited to rock band dinning and bad news droned between commercial breaks. Actually, radio has probably never been so diversified. FM frequencies supply hours of all kinds of music, often uninterrupted, and are well worth dialing about to locate.

## HEALTHY WAYS TO RELEASE TENSION

The quotation that began this chapter admonished the reader against "being grieved and taking all matters to heart." The almost overwhelming impacts of the artificial stressors and affectors of modern life are now believed to extract very high penalties from men and women who submit themselves to conditions at work and at home that cause deep, powerful reactions which they bottle up inside their bodies and minds. The offices of cardiologists and psychiatrists are jammed with dollar-driven, clock-chasing, achievement-motivated adults and young people severely damaged by inappropriate diet and lack of exercise whose lives are endangered by the bombardment of urban stimuli from the outside and willed or unconscious physical responses to stress and strain from the inside. These people believe they should not "get angry and shout at times." They are concerned by what others will think of them, worried that employers or competitors will observe emotional responses and interpret them as weaknesses. Anger, aggression, and ambition can combine to create a compulsive and self-destructive life pattern. A certain amount of roaring and arm-waving releases these tensions, but the urban executive on the rise is as self-inhibited as he is self-propelled.

### "Type A" and "Type B" Behavior

Although not without their critics, Drs. Rosenman and Friedman have classified this observable behavior as "Type A." Type B personalities are markedly less combative, capable of relaxing as they work, and much less given to violent mood swings. These two groups of men, both living in an ideally stimulating temperate region, San Francisco, ate the same sort of too-rich diet, exercised only sporadically and smoked about the same amount. Type A men suffered 600% more heart attacks than the group described as Type B.

Laboratory analysis of blood samples indicated to Rosenman and Friedman that superstimulated adult males experienced stress responses with abnormally high levels of adrenaline and norepinephrine. Observation supported by chemical data tends to be taken seriously, even by skeptical or envious researchers in the same field. The important book by Friedman and Rosenman, now available in paperback, can be obtained from local bookstores, where it is well-known as "Type A Behavior."

Readers of Friedman and Rosenman will observe that their last chapter urges retraining of many daily habits and attitudes. It is actually a guided program to restore the "Type A" personality to a more normal and natural daily existence. Hopefully, the general advice given here will have positive, preventive effects that will enable heedful readers to avoid the "Type A" syndrome. It is easier, cheaper, and safer to exercise self-control than to restore a victim of self-tyranny. It is more health-sustaining to ancitipate and to avoid than to calm and to cure. To a large extent, ill health is an accident depending on the proclivity and susceptibility of the host. While human body weather can be profoundly affected by the impacts of the modern environment, better body weather can be made and maintained by a prudent embracing of those elemental forces that shape the natural environment.

Any man who lived more than one hundred years of active life is worth listening to. You may recall that Cornaro over three centuries ago urged "a kind of regimen into which every man may put himself without interruption to business, expense of money or loss of time." While he held that "medicines are indeed absolutely necessary in acute distempers," he favored temperance and exercise "to make luxury consistent with health." We have some simple ways of deflecting or reducing those impacts and abuses that affect and stress the human body and that are contemporaneous with modern, urbanized technologies.

Man has been conditioned by his natural environment for untold hundreds of thousands of years. His creation of new conveniences and comforts has been of enormous benefit to him as a producer and consumer. He appears, however, to have paid a price for progress, and the penalties are greatest when he forfeits self-regulation for profit and permits his own creations to determine how he lives. These pages considering the health impacts of natural and man-made weather are intended to promote better body weather, reversing Cornaro's words, "to make health consistent with luxury."

# Bibliography

Adams, Ruth. *Did You Ever See a Fat Squirrel?* Emmaus, Pa.: Rodale Press, 1973.

Carruthers, Malcolm. *The Western Way of Death.* New York: Pantheon Books, 1974.

Cheraskin, E., and Ringsdorf, W. M. *Psychodietetics.* New York: Stein & Day, 1974.

Cousteau, Jacques-Yves, and Cousteau, Philippe. *The Shark.* New York: Doubleday & Co., 1970.

Dempsey, David. "Noise." *New York Times Magazine,* 23 November 1975.

Diehl, Harold S., and Dalrymple, W. *Healthful Living.* New York: Mc-Graw-Hill Book Co., 1973.

Duberman, Martin. "The Case of the Gay Sergeant." *New York Times Magazine,* 9 November 1975.

Esser, Aristide H. "Environment and Mental Health." In *Science, Medicine and Man,* vol. 1, edited by Thomas McEwen, pp. 181–93. Elmsford, N.Y.: Pergamon Press, 1974.

173

# Bibliography

Friedman, Meyer, and Rosenman, Ray H. *Type A Behavior and Your Heart*. New York: Alfred Knopf, 1974.

Goodman, Louis S., and Gilman, Alfred, eds. *The Pharmacological Basis of Therapeutics*. 4th ed. New York: Macmillan Co. 1970.

Griffiths, Joel, and Ballantine, Richard. *Silent Slaughter*. Chicago: Henry Regnery Co., 1972.

*Health Consequences of Sulfur Oxides*. Research Triangle Park, N.C.: U.S. Environmental Protection Agency, 1974.

Hillman, W. S. "Injury of Tomato Plants by Continuous Light, etc." *American Journal of Botany* 43 (1956): 89.

Huntington, E. *Season of Birth: Its Relation to Human Abilities*. New York: John Wiley, 1938.

Lewis, Howard R., and Lewis, Martha E. *Psychosomatics*. New York: Viking Press, 1972.

Linde, Shirley Motter, and Finnerty, Frank, Jr. *High Blood Pressure*. New York: David McKay Co., 1975.

Luce, Gay Gaer. *Biological Rhythms in Psychiatry and Medicine*. Washington, D.C.: U.S. Department of Health, Education and Welfare and the National Institute of Mental Health, 1970.

*Metropolitan Life Insurance Company Statistical Bulletin* 55 (January 1974): 4-6, and (February 1974): 5-7.

Mills, Clarence A. *Medical Climatology*. Springfield, Ill.: Charles C. Thomas Co., 1939.

Ott, John N. *Health and Light*. Old Greenwich, Conn.: Devin-Adair Co., 1973.

Pilgrim, Ira. *The Topic of Cancer*. New York: Thomas Y. Crowell Co., 1974.

Pinckney, Edward R., and Pinckney, Cathy. *The Cholesterol Controversy*. Los Angeles: Sherbourne Press, 1973.

Reuben, David. *The Save Your Life Diet*. New York: Random House, 1975.

Rodale, J. I. *Your Diet and Your Heart*. Emmaus, Pa.: Rodale Press, 1969.

Rodale, Robert. *The Best Health Ideas I Know*. Emmaus, Pa.: Rodale Press, 1974.

Rosenberg, Harold, and Feldzamen, A. N. *The Doctor's Book of Vitamin Therapy*. New York: G. P. Putnam's Sons, 1974.

Tromp, S. W., and Weihe, W. H., eds. *Biometeorology*, vol. 2, parts 1 and 2. Proceedings of the 3d International Biometeorological Congress held at Pau, France. Elmsford, N.Y.: Pergamon Press, 1967.

―――. *Biometeorology*, vol. 3. Proceedings of the 4th International Biometeorological Congress held at Rutgers University, New Brunswick, N.J. Amsterdam: Swets & Zeitlinger, N.V., 1967.

*174*

————. *Biometeorology*, vol. 4, parts 1 and 2. Proceedings of the 5th International Biometeorological Congress held at Montreux, Switzerland. Amsterdam: Swets & Zeitlinger, N.V., 1970.

Watson, Lyall. *Super Nature*. New York: Bantam Books, 1974.

Zohman, Lenore R., and Tobias, Jerome S. *Cardiac Rehabilitation*. New York and London: Grune and Stratton, 1970.

# Index

**178**